The Habit Switch

How Little Changes Can Produce Massive Results for Your Health, Diet and Energy Levels by Introducing Incremental Mini Habits

ROMNEY NELSON

The Habit Switch

This book is dedicated in memory of my step-father John. He was such a supportive father that departed for heaven far too early. We miss you greatly Johnny Pops.

TABLE OF CONTENTS

INTRODUCTION

How amazing would it be if it was as simple as flicking a switch to suddenly change your health and fitness habits for good! What if this was possible? What if it required just small daily changes to your current lifestyle, rather than radical changes that are unlikely to have a long term and positive impact?

What I'm about to show you will prove that with just small and incremental daily changes and the right systems, *you can* transform your health and fitness habits for good, but on one condition.... you must switch your mindset from short term to long term thinking.

Welcome to The Habit Switch. My name is Romney Nelson, and I want to provide you with all the knowledge to help make a transformation with how you view your fitness and health.

To provide you with some details of my background, I have a significant wealth of experience in health, fitness and wellbeing. I have a

Bachelor of Physical Education & Health, and I have been Head of Faculty for some of the leading Independent Schools in Australia and the UK. I am a qualified Personal Trainer and coach, I have represented Australia at the World Championships in Hong Kong for Dragon Boat Racing and have participated in the National Championships for Surf Life Saving.

I have complimented my sporting achievements with an extensive employment career. I have served on several Executive Teams and National positions of responsibility. I have worked for the Australian Football League (AFL) and currently have a seat on the Advisory Board of Australia's largest mobile dental provider with over 40,000 patients per year. My personal experience in the fields of health, exercise physiology and sports training has provided me with the opportunity to share all that I have learned to help you regain control over your eating habits and physical fitness.

I wrote The Habit Switch with a key focus to guide you through the methods to build the right systems, structures and mindset to help you determine what advice is real and what advice is pure marketing in the billion-dollar fitness and dieting industry.

Further to this, *The Habit Switch* will provide you with all the information that will enable you to significantly improve your diet, health and fitness in a simplified and easy to implement system.

We gravitate towards books that will help us.

There's a reason why you are reading this book and it's because we all want to improve our diet and fitness to keep ourselves healthy, but it seems like every day there is a new article with an entirely different way to go about it. It is easy to have the best intentions when starting a new diet routine but still find yourself falling victim to confusing marketing practices that are only trying to achieve short-term success without caring if their methods are effective for the long term.

Diet and exercise plans that help you lose a few pounds very quickly are effective in the short term, but they often lose steam the longer you follow them. Some diets are simply too restrictive to follow for more than a few weeks, leaving you lethargic, hungry and craving something more substantial, ultimately leading you towards ending the diet. Other diet plans ask for a significant commitment of time and combining this with very busy lives; they tend to fall by the wayside. Dropping an exercise plan or not getting the right results on a diet can make you feel unnecessarily guilty, but the truth is, the lack of success on these plans is due to the focus on the short term rather than more powerful and lasting long-term results.

Additionally, due to the abundance of different diet plans, health and fitness advice from various sources can often vary greatly. The information these sources suggest can even contradict other fitness books and articles, leaving you uncertain about what will really work to improve your health. One study will claim that frequent alcohol consumption leads to health problems, while another will tell you to have a glass of red wine every day. Some sources tell you to eat more fat, while others suggest you to stop eating fat altogether. The same is true for whether or not you should be eating red meat and incorporating designated 'superfoods' into your diet. Even health suggestions that are not contradictory can become overwhelming due to the sheer number of factors you must keep track of. Altering your diet, counting your steps, reducing your calories, keeping track of macros, drinking more water, and dozens of other measures ask for an unrealistically significant contribution of your time and energy, which can be especially frustrating when you see minimal results even after all of that work. With all of this in mind, it is no surprise that it is hard to narrow down precisely what you should and shouldn't be doing to get and stay healthy. But what is the solution to cutting through all the confusion and figuring out what works?

Improving your health needs to become natural, and you need to feel comfortable with the process. Adopting a diet and exercise regimen that benefits your body and mind is instead a gradual process of improving your daily habits and allowing them to build incrementally to create real change.

Healthy Habits

Habits are the little actions we take every day, even without thinking about them, that make up our daily routines. Small habits can have a surprisingly large impact on your life. Their strength lies in the fact that they promote constant action in your subconscious, letting you break down a difficult task into more manageable segments and complete it over a length of time. For example, say you want to write a novel. Trying to write thousands of words each day would certainly be a formidable task. However, if you simply committed yourself to write a mere 200 words a day, a habit which fits more easily into your schedule, you would make progress on your book every day. The act of writing would become habitual over time, and with steady progress, you would finish your book much sooner than you once thought possible. Habits can be applied to every part of your life, including health and fitness, and making good use of them can yield amazing results.

Adopting healthy habits means leaving behind unhealthy ones. These bad habits likely started small with minimal impact on your physical fitness, but over time they grew to become serious problems. One white chocolate and blueberry muffin on occasions is not a big deal, but when that muffin turns into one every day, it becomes a bad habit that can prevent you from getting healthier. Weight gain can be a product of just a small amount of excess calories over a long period of time. However, just as small negative habits can cause health problems, small diet changes and increases in physical activity can keep you from gaining weight and counteract the effects of unhealthy behaviors. In either case, your health is not a product of single decisions but rather the sum of all of your habits over time. The solution that is most effective for weight loss then, is starting small and reversing the negative habits you have picked up over the years.

Small, constructive habits have more long-term benefits than attempting to change everything about your lifestyle all at once. Trying to make too great of a change in a short period is likely to lead to exhaustion and a loss of willpower, leaving you right back where you started. Instead, try introducing habits that are easy to complete and don't take up too much of your time. These easily manageable tasks let you make progress on your goals while also training your brain to practice healthy habits each day. Once you are comfortable with the initial habits, you can slowly build upon them. You will find the success you are looking for without the concern of not being able to keep up because you overloaded yourself too early. Once you adopt good habits, improving your health becomes as easy as flipping 'The Habit Switch'.

Flipping the switch

This book will teach you how to flip the switch and turn on positive healthy habits. The first step of your new health solution is a four-part process called STOP>REVIEW>PIVOT and POWER. This system allows you to stop and evaluate your current habits, review the progress or lack of improvement of your current situation, pivot your habits towards those that will help you achieve your goals, and then power through to success. The right mindset is also critical to ensuring the decisions you make today will positively impact your health tomorrow.

The Habit Switch will provide you with:

- An understanding of the powerful Stop, Review, Pivot, and Power system
- Tips for establishing a mindset of positivity and focus
- Specific, actionable steps and mini habits you can implement that, when compounded over time, lead to exponential benefits for your diet, fitness, and energy levels.
- The reason why "no pain, no gain" is wrong and how you can achieve incredible long-term gains by flipping the switch on this mentality.

- An appreciation that the role of exercise and supportive eating habits can have for a long term and sustainable approach.

You can achieve change without any of the difficulties associated with extreme dieting, excessive exercise and adjusting your lifestyle too quickly. All it takes is a series of small steps and the dedication to make a change in your life.

With *The Habit Switch,* you can completely revolutionize your mindset through the development and implementation of mini habits. You will learn how so many people have been manipulated by marketing in the fitness industry. You will also learn why it's time to introduce a sensible and bulletproof strategy for mastering your health habits, starting with incremental changes and leading to huge changes in your life.

Implementing the mini habits introduced to you in this book will unlock lifelong positive changes. You can experience higher levels of energy, have greater productivity, maintain a healthy body weight, and become knowledgeable about behaviors and foods that are healthy for your mind as well as your body. The daily exercise and fitness habits you develop will be long-term and sustainable, not just shortcuts and quick fix changes that are likely to fall apart under pressure. The changes you will be encouraged to make through daily habits will really stick.

You have spent enough time searching through endless diet and exercise plans that never get you the results you deserve. *The Habit Switch* is the resource you have been waiting for. It will provide you with a sustainable approach that doesn't stop at short-term results but rather, will yield long-term success. It is time to start making changes and adopting habits that will help you become the best version of yourself, and it all starts with you. The decisions you make and the actions you take will lead you down the path to living a happier, healthier and more fulfilling life.

I think it is time that you are provided with a no-nonsense and honest guide that isn't full of shortcuts promising changes in 7 days, rather, a book that provides actionable steps that can be implemented over time that will build the foundation for long term success. You must be open to change, and it begins with a commitment to taking small steps now that will result in giant leaps later on.

Chapter 1

<u>My Habits</u>

The Mindset and Systems for a Healthy Body

Changing your daily habits is a powerful tool, but it can be difficult to know where to start. When figuring out which habits you should prioritize to improve your health, it is helpful to have an example of a good set of habits. I want to provide you with my personal list of habits that I do every day to ensure I am making progress towards my goals. I believe that supplying you with this information will give you a template to base your habits off and help you define what you want to achieve and the way you want to achieve it. Everyone's individual habits are going to be different; your daily habits should be reflective of what you value, what you want to improve, and the time you can commit to each goal. By sharing my habits, I hope to guide you through the process I used to select my own habits and show how they each support my endeavors.

My personal mantra is "What can I do today that will further my personal growth and move me closer to reaching my full potential tomorrow?" Every day should bring you closer to reaching your potential. As you will find out as you read this book, I don't advocate for perfectionism, but rather personal fulfilment. You should strive to become the best possible version of yourself, not someone else. This means following your own dreams, not the goals someone else has set for you. As a result, I develop my habits based on my personal goals because they are made up of the things that I want for myself and my family. This includes my physical health as well as my mental well-being. Our bodies are the vehicles we need to achieve all of our goals, so we owe it to ourselves to look after the gift and opportunity we have been given.

How I Established My Habit Schedule

My habit schedule is influenced by who I am as a person. People who know me well appreciate that I am well-structured, organized and very focused. I also consider myself to be committed to the goals I set for myself. As a result, I schedule my habits with the aim to do them at the same time every day. Having a schedule to fall back on reinforces positive behaviors and helps me keep track of my progress. Because of this, I have scheduled my habits in a way that allows me to maximize their benefits and give them an appropriate amount of time. I make sure to avoid rushing a new or developing habit so that it "takes root" firmly and develops correctly. I try to take each action seriously and give them time to develop incrementally so that I don't overwhelm myself.

My diet is one area that I pay careful attention to. A healthy, nutritious diet provides me with the energy I need to accomplish all of my other goals, so I need to ensure I am keeping myself in the best possible shape. I would consider my diet to be well balanced, mainly as a result of my upbringing, my background in sports, and my qualifications in physical education and health. I always want to embody what I suggest for others. If I encourage others to eat certain foods and maintain a balanced diet or to exercise a certain way, it's because I do it myself. Of course, I also think it is important to highlight that I do still drift on occasions from a diet of nutritious foods. I still have the occasional pizza, a beer with family and friends, a good coffee, and even a great muffin. These little treats can be nice to enjoy now and then. However, I try to keep them to a minimum in my diet. My personal eating habits restrict less healthy foods to around five percent of my overall diet. This leaves plenty of room for more nutritious options most days, which bring me closer to my goals of living a long and healthy life. I fill the rest of my diet with healthy foods that provide my body with the fuel I need to take me to my 100th birthday. Exercise is another important part of my routine. It is a habit that I picked up when I was younger while training for competitive sports, which also left me with a few niggling injuries. I am lucky that only one, a bulging disk in my neck from a gymnastics injury, impacts my mobility on occasions so that I can do most physical exercises. However, I recognize that this is not true for everyone and that as we age, exercise becomes about finding sustainable activities we can integrate into our lives without increasing the chance of injury. Many friends of mine who have sustained injuries during competitive sports and long-distance running do have limitations with their mobility. When finding the right exercise for you, it is critical to take into account your limitations and choose something you can do on a regular basis.

Ultimately, my habits are structured to provide long-term support and assistance on my journey to reach my goals, which is the same idea you should take into account when deciding on your own habits. I will expand on the methods I use to narrow down the habits that best suit my lifestyle throughout the book, as well as how I began implementing these habits and building them incrementally so they can build up to compounding effects over time. However, I want to provide a word of warning first. The habits that work well for me may not be suitable for you. I am using my personal schedule in the book primarily to illustrate the power of habits and what they allow you to do, not to suggest you copy my habits directly. They are suited to my own long-term goals, but they may not be reflective of yours. Spend some time thinking about what you want to achieve and how you would be able to go about achieving it as you create your own list of daily supportive habits.

My Morning Routine

Detailing every single habit I do each day would take a great deal of time, so I have limited my scope to just my morning routine, which I hope serves as an introduction and a template for your own. Use it to get an idea of my structure and how I have been able to incorporate ten healthy and supportive habits over 2 hours.

- **4:25 AM** - Wake up
- **4:30 AM** - Power walk with my dog and listen to an educational podcast
- **5:05 AM** - Drink 500 mL water and take one magnesium supplement
- **5:07 AM** - Breakfast of porridge with fresh fruit and one scoop of natural yoghurt
- **5:16 AM** - 120 push-ups (4 sets of 30)
- **5:20 AM** - 200 sit-ups (4 sets of 50)
- **5:30 AM** - Personal daily goal affirmations (recorded and played back)
- **5:35 AM** - Meditation and visualization for 15 minutes
- **5:50 AM** - The Daily Goal Tracker: record what I'm grateful for, my current thoughts, and three key actions
- **6:00 AM** – Shower
- **6:15 AM** - Reading for 20 minutes
- **6:35 AM** - Begin the day

These habits are short activities that take up a small portion of my day. They are not too difficult for me to complete, which means I have no trouble repeating them each morning. Over the course of one month, assuming I do these habits six days a week and use Sunday as my rest and recovery day, they build up to a powerful transformation. Here is the massive compounding impact I receive by the end of the month:

- Walking/exercise = **12 hrs.**
- Podcasts (inspirational interviews) = **12 hrs.**
- Push-ups = **2,880** push-ups for upper body strength and tone
- Sit-ups = **4,800** sit-ups for core strength and avoiding lower back pain
- Planting my goals subconsciously via daily affirmations = **2 hrs.**
- Meditation/visualization = **8 hrs.**
- Prioritization of daily activities to move closer to my goals = **72** key actions
- Journaling six things I am grateful for daily = **24** days of journaling
- Reading = **8 hrs.**

You can now see just how much of an impact mini habits can have on your life. If I simply decided to do 4,800 sit-ups in a month without any other planning, I would likely end up slacking some days and failing to reach my goal. By breaking the process up into more bite-sized, easily achievable sections each day, I have no trouble reaching my goal. I hope that you can use this process of establishing mini habits to achieve the same levels of tremendous change and amazing results for your health, diet, and energy levels.

Chapter 2

Compound Growth

+

Mini Habits = Big Impact

Part one of *The Habit Switch* is all about transformation. How is transformation possible, what sort of mindset do you need to adopt to encourage change, and how will you devise your plan to improve your life? Understanding the habit switch process will help you answer all of these questions.

This section will help you begin to identify the areas you want to improve in that matter to you personally. You should always work towards goals that you care about rather than what is expected of you; doing so will provide the necessary motivation to keep up with your new schedule. The section will also discuss the benefits you can see if you stick to mini habits over a long period of time, which can build to amazing results that would have felt near-impossible to tackle all at once. With the power of small changes, you can completely turn your health and fitness around.

Part of making changes is developing a plan that will take you from your first steps all the way to your goals. By identifying where you want to end up, you can establish the steps you will take to keep you on the right track, aligned with your values, and turning negative habits into positive ones. Great goal setting, aided by my method of DR. ACTION™, will help you organize your habits in a way that encourages you to always keep moving forward and keeps you from faltering on your path to success. But before you can do that, you must understand what it takes to make a transformative change.

What Does It Take to Transform?

Changing your mindset is the key to changing your life. The wrong mindset can keep you stuck in the same situation for months or even years, unable to make changes that stick despite your best intentions. The right mindset, on the other hand, can make you see every opportunity the universe throws your way in a new light. It will help you develop confidence and maintain your commitment to reaching success. Mindset then is imperative to a real transformation.

There has been a great deal of research into the different kinds of mindset, and one school of thought is that of the static mindset and the development mindset. Static mindset suggests that you are predisposed towards certain qualities, through your nature or some other innate skill, and the things you can excel in are for the most part set in stone. A development mindset, on the other hand, means you believe you can grow and expand your skills with effort and experience. While the static mindset can allow you to improve in certain areas, it suggests that you are not capable of improving in all areas, or those that you do not initially excel at. This means it can be harder to change bad habits and try new things, as you believe you simply cannot get any better if you don't show an immediate aptitude for something. A static mindset attempts to dissuade you from change.

A development mindset promotes attempting new things, possibly failing but always showing improvement with each step of your journey. In short, it encourages moving forward and branching out. This is what makes a development mindset so powerful. When you believe you are capable of getting better at a task or activity, you will give yourself more time to keep pushing at something that is difficult for you rather than giving up when your first attempts do not lead to success. You can allow yourself to find the fitness habits that work for you and avoid falling into the trap of thinking that if you do not see instant results, you will never see them.

If you currently operate under a static mindset, start shifting your thoughts over to a development mindset instead. You can accomplish this through a few different ways, the first of which involves accepting the possibility of failure. Remember that no failure needs to be permanent and that faltering can give us the experience and tools we need to succeed. Additionally, you can start to prioritize the journey of growth over the destination. While you always want to be moving towards your goals, there is a lot to enjoy in the process of improving as well, so don't forget to celebrate the little milestones along the way. It is also essential to keep the reasons why you are seeking change in the forefront of your mind. Research suggests that people with development mindsets have a greater sense of purpose, which allows them to maintain focus on the big picture (Briggs, 2015, para. 18). Your sense of purpose, or the reason why you are committed to your goals, will ensure you stick to your habits and successfully transform yourself.

What is transformation?

What does it mean to transform your life, not just make minor tweaks and alterations? What separates a temporary, unsustainable burst of movement from something more permanent? To know the difference, you need to have a good idea of what transformation is and what it is not. Cambridge Dictionary's definition of the word transformational is "able to produce a big change or improvement in a situation" (Cambridge Dictionary, n.d., para. 2). Let's break this definition down into its parts to get a better understanding.

Firstly, something that is transformational is "able," not guaranteed, to produce a change. It may be very likely that a given action, like eating less junk food or doing a few extra sit-ups, will contribute to better health. However, it is not a guarantee if the rest of your habits do not support the change. This is why it is so vital to ensure all of your daily habits are supportive and that you stick to your supportive habits as often as you can.

Transformational actions are likely to lead to a "big change or improvement," not a minimal one. Losing two or three pounds is not much of a transformation, but committing yourself to improve your health is a full-body change that qualifies as a large-scale improvement. To make a transformation, you need to be ready to make lasting changes in the areas that matter.

Finally, transformations involve changes to your "situation." To expand on this, I'm referring to where you are at currently regarding your mental attitude and physical wellbeing. A real transformation incites change in every aspect of your life. The *STOP>REVIEW>PIVOT* and *POWER* system discussed in later chapters will show you how to assess your current situation and set you off in the direction of improving all areas of importance to you. Remember that your goal is for these changes in your situation to be permanent. To make a lasting change, it is not enough to spend just one week on a crash diet and expect the change to stick. You need to make a long-term commitment to establishing and cultivating new habits.

Making a Long-Term Commitment

Making a lasting healthy change takes time. It is all too tempting to believe that once you start adopting a healthy diet and exercising, that everything will just fall into place. It takes a long-term commitment to change, and a never quit attitude that will provide the results that you desire. If you want to improve, you must accept that a long-lasting change in your health is a product of slow changes over time rather than drastic, unsustainable changes.

Expecting results to occur too quickly can be harmful to your long-term success. It can even point to a subconscious desire to sabotage yourself and give yourself an excuse to give up on extremely strict, difficult diets. Looking for instant change "is a mechanism to make it easy for you to give up. If you know that you have to do something, which is not possible, then you know that it is doomed to fail" (Heijligers, n.d., para. 9) and you can simply quit. You give yourself the excuse to give up because you have created an impossible expectation for yourself. This can mean that no change ever occurs. If you give yourself time to set up a good foundation instead of constantly looking for results, you will be more likely to stick with your fitness plan for as long as it takes those results to appear.

You may also be operating under the belief that if you do not see the change right away, nothing is working. Many diets boast that you can lose five pounds (2kgs) in the first week, or twenty pounds (9 kgs) in twenty days, therefore you go into all diet plans expecting to see immediate results. If you don't see what you expect, this may cause you to drop the diet altogether. In reality, a large portion of lasting change is setting up the groundwork for future benefits. While you may not see immediate results, that does not mean nothing is happening; you are giving yourself the tools to succeed in the future.

Investing in Your Future

The single best investment you can make is in yourself. You need a healthy mind and body that will allow you to achieve everything you desire. Set goals, keep yourself healthy, expand your knowledge, and ultimately be aware of your value. Knowing your knowledge and actions matter is an investment in your morale (Tull, 2017, para. 9). Remaining self-confident and positive will help you keep going when it would be much easier to give up. Consider what matters most to you, and what are the specific outcomes you are hoping to achieve? Forget what other people want you to do and the expectations they place on you and just consider your desires. In particular, think about the long-term goals that each step of the dieting and exercise process will help you to achieve and select steps that fit your end goals.

The idea of deriving habits from self-defined goals is well-researched and supported in many areas of healthcare. In 2012, Gardner, Lally & Wardle found that if doctors helped patients set their own health goals, it actually supported patients' sense of autonomy and sustained their interest.

Steve Jobs, the co-founder of Apple, summarized it well when he said; "*Your time is limited, so don't waste it living someone else's life. Don't be trapped by dogma – which is living with the results of other people's thinking. Don't let the noise of other's opinions drown out your inner voice. And most important, have the courage to follow your heart and intuition. They somehow already know what you truly want to become. Everything else is secondary.*"

Healthy Habit Change
Why Small Is Actually BIG!

Big changes can come from relatively small actions. It would be impossible to completely uproot every behavior pattern you have subconsciously followed for years in a single day. Think of your journey as laying a garden path made of pavers. You will need to lay one paver at a time as this will allow the next paver to fit to create your pattern. You will start slow, ensuring you have a solid foundation to build from. As you lay more pavers, it becomes easier, your momentum builds, and your skills grow. So, start with the first paver - that is, begin laying the foundation for your health overhaul with small habits that will eventually lead to a considerable change in behavior.

Habits are so small that they often go unnoticed unless you are consciously looking for them. You may perform a bad habit, like grabbing a takeaway iced coffee with lunch every day without thinking twice about it. The problem comes when these small actions build-up, and without realizing it, you have had an iced coffee every day for months or years at a time. The solution involves exchanging these bad habits for good ones and conditioning yourself to develop a different response to the same stimulus.

Your surroundings and environment also have a considerable influence on your actions. Being in a particular location, seeing the clock hit a specific time of day, and taking a certain action can all be triggers for different habits. Every time you encounter stimulus A, you perform action B. This behavior, carried out over a period of time, is how a habit is formed. Even the act of brushing your teeth after the stimulus of waking up in the morning is a habit that has been cultivated over years of practice. When you get into the habit of making the right choice after encountering a given stimulus, you will start to make that choice subconsciously every time. This leads to a compounding effect that will allow you to see stunning results as time goes on.

I need to highlight that changing your habits does take time. If you want to achieve sustainable success, not just a burst of change that fades after a brief period, you need to let time take its course. The changes you are making now can appear very small at first, but if you repeat that behavior over an extended period, these supportive habits add up to be life-changing.

James Clear in his bestselling book Atomic Habits articulated it well by saying that habits "seem to make little difference on any given day and yet the impact they deliver over the months and years can be enormous. It is only when looking back two, five, or perhaps ten years later that the value of good habits and the cost of bad ones becomes strikingly apparent". The important part of this step is to realize that you are developing habits that support a healthy future, which means they must be given time to compound into big differences.

Many people are experts at negative compounding, where small negative choices repeated over vast periods of time add up to a net negative. Poor habit development leads them to get in the way of their ability to achieve their goals. Negative compounding can be just as powerful as its positive counterpart but in the opposite direction. To stop compounding negative habits, focus on turning those habits into positive ones.

Positive compounding uses a similar theory to achieve the opposite effect. It involves the introduction of tiny, one percent difference changes in daily behaviors that get amplified over time. In positive compounding, "things add up. You learn one skill. Then another. You finish one project. Then another. Over time, your accomplishments add up to form an impressive feat" (Foroux, n.d., para. 14). The trick is not to get caught up in failing to see immediate results in 30, 60, or even 90 days, reverting back to poor choices, and losing your momentum. Real compounding can take much longer to get going, but it is worth it for the incredible success you can use it to achieve. When setting your long-term goals, think about those that can be accomplished over no less than five years. That may seem like a very long time, but if you want results that last, you need to be thinking long term. That way, even if introducing the habit takes you 90 days, the initial time to implement that habit will be minuscule compared to the positive impact over the next 1800 days or more. The problem that many people face is that they try and take drastic leaps in a short period. Remember, you only need to make incremental changes and let them build and this will offer a life-time change and impact, not just a short-term solution.

Incremental Introduction

It is an essential stage of 'The Habit Switch' to break down the process of how to put a new habit into action, and this is by introducing it incrementally as you would now expect. To provide you with a clear example, let us assume that you currently rise at 7:00 AM, but you would like to get up at 6:20 AM so that you can add in an extra 30 minutes of reading in your day. Merely setting the alarm for 6:20 AM and trying to change your schedule with no build-up preparation is likely to get you hitting the snooze button, which could lead to you accidentally sleeping in even later than your usual time. If you take the time to wake up five minutes earlier every few days incrementally, something that takes much less willpower will easily allow you to reach 6:20 AM with minimal effort or impact on your alertness or energy levels.

I have used this example to great effect in my previous book 'Magnetic Goals'. In the example I offer the following strategy;

Start by initially setting your alarm five minutes earlier every third day, six days per week, with Sunday being a day when you can sleep in. The schedule shows how a small change every three days would play out, allowing you five minutes to get out of bed and perhaps make a cup of tea before beginning to read.

- **Week 1**, Mon/Tues/Weds: 6:55 AM alarm, no reading at this stage.
- **Week 1**, Thurs/Fri/Sat: Alarm is wound back by 5 minutes to 6:50 AM. Still no reading at this stage.
- **Week 2**, Mon/Tues/Weds: 6:45 AM alarm, 10 minutes of reading commences

- **Week 2**, Thurs/Fri/Sat: Alarm is brought back to 6:40 AM alarm, permitting 15 minutes of reading
- **Week 3**, Mon/Tues/Weds: 6:35 AM alarm, 20 minutes of reading
- **Week 3**, Thurs/Fri/Sat: Alarm is brought back to 6:30 AM alarm, permitting 25 minutes of reading
- **Week 4**, Mon/Tues/Weds: 6:25 AM alarm, 30 minutes of reading
- **Week 4**, Thurs/Fri/Sat: Alarm is brought back to 6:20 AM alarm, permitting you to reach you goal of 35 minutes of reading

In just 30 days, you have shifted your schedule to achieve a 6:20 AM start to your day, and you have accumulated over two hours of reading in the process. This is great, but the biggest change will now start to compound, now that you have extra time in your schedule to read.

Over one year, you will have an extra 40 minutes in your schedule, six days a week, 52 weeks a year, totaling an extra 208hrs in your schedule. This is the equivalent of adding 8 ½ additional days to your year. If you can keep this up for five years, you can achieve 1,032 extra hours or 43 days you did not have access to before. Trust me; you won't miss the

40 minutes of sleep each day in the face of the significant benefits you will receive. Being able to read hundreds of books you would have otherwise missed out on can produce amazing, substantial changes in your life and improve your skills and knowledge.

Blocking Out Temptation

Healthy habit change will help you avoid the bad habits you might otherwise engage in and develop a blind spot for the things that would have otherwise caught your eye. When you eat junk food regularly, especially sugary foods, you tend to seek them out and crave them. Once you cut down on your consumption, seeing junk food does not tempt you quite as much as it once did. For example, grocery and convenience stores tend to place sugary items like confectionary near the check-out aisle, so they catch your eye as you wait for your turn. Harmful eating habits that result in a dependency on sugar create attractions to these items and increase the likelihood you will buy one on your way out. Once you develop healthy eating habits, these items seem to all but disappear from your vision. They become much easier to ignore, to the point that I rarely notice them at all now, as they rest firmly in my blind spot.

Healthy habits aren't just limited to diet. They also involve exercise and small changes to improve your exercise schedule over time will provide huge benefits in the long run. Where most people get it wrong is by trying to do too much and make significant changes in short periods of time. By doing this, you risk burning yourself out and not having the energy you need to get your healthy, incremental exercise done each day. If you skip the slow adjustment process and dive right in, you can end up feeling sore, nauseous, develop discomfort, risk an injury, or have reduced motivation to stick to your plan. This is why the incremental approach is so valuable.

The Marketing Geniuses – Avoiding the Lure of the Diet and Fitness Fad

Top marketers at big companies are pros at guiding public opinion. Food marketing, in particular, is a large industry that makes up everything from dairy to produce junk food like chips and cookies. It is sometimes hard to settle in for a movie without first walking by the bright lights advertising the bucket of popcorn or the choc tops or even the extra-large soft drinks all reduced to a special price just for movie go'ers. Still, you know that these kinds of foods are okay as occasional treats but aren't healthy for you in the long run. While you may occasionally give into the temptation to enjoy a handful of popcorn, you know that all the butter and salt isn't doing you any favors.

The same cannot always be said for food marketing that masquerades as health tips. Unfortunately, there is a lot of conflicting advice about what you should and shouldn't be eating to stay healthy. Most people agree that having a slice of cake every day isn't a healthy choice, but opinions differ when it comes to things like meat consumption, fats, and carbs. What is healthy on one diet may be disallowed entirely on another. Keep a sharp eye out for any claims that seem to come from smart marketing rather than an honest portrayal of eating the right foods and in correct proportions.

Many companies try to dress up their products as 'healthier' alternatives to the more standard versions, and while this may technically be true, this doesn't always mean they are healthy. A slice of cake is healthier than the whole cake, but it is still packed with sugar and butter. Keep in mind that just because something is technically healthier than its alternative, that does not mean it is healthy or that you should eat it regularly. For example, light beer or low carb beer may be considered healthier than full-strength beer, but it's not nearly as good for you as water would be in the equivalent amounts, and the consumption of light beer can still lead to similar health concerns as full-strength beer if you consume too many. A product that is lower in fats or sugars than another may only be lower by a gram or two, even though they claim "lower fat" would lead most people to believe the difference is more drastic than that. Some marketing will also use various spelling variations like 'Lite Sour Cream' or use stats to confuse you; for example 20% less fat. You should then ask, 20% less fat than what? If it is 20% less fat now, what was it beforehand? It is important to always have a critical eye for marketing practices that try to capitalize on health trends so that you can identify the truly helpful advice from the fakes.

Similar technically true but misleading claims can be seen in fitness workout plans. Pay special attention to buzzwords meant to draw your attention without crossing the boundary into being misleading. To give an example of this in the exercise industry, how often have you seen the word *unsurpassed* thrown around? Would this imply that it is significantly better than the alternatives, without being misleading? Something like "unsurpassed" suggests that a program is better than all other alternatives, when in reality it may be just about the same, or even slightly worse with no official measurements comparing the two programs. Always remain cautious and assume that if something sounds too good to be true, it just might be, especially when it comes to health and fitness trends and the growing market that is worth billions of dollars annually.

The Troubles with Trends

The health and fitness market has recently become especially profitable as more people look for healthy alternatives to their typical patterns and prioritize getting in shape. In the last decade, "there's been a 108% increase in the healthy eating and nutrition market to $276.5 billion, and a 78% increase in personalized health to $243 billion," so to call the industry booming might be an understatement (Settembre, 2018, para. 13). While helpful advice is always welcome, certain fitness trends are less about providing reliable advice and more about providing a short-term solution that will ensure their product or service with notoriety. Be wary of trends that are more focused on marketing than concrete, actionable advice.

Trends are by their very nature temporary booms, which does not speak well to their effectiveness in the long term. They tend to focus on weekly or even daily results instead of considering the importance of long-term achievements. Remember that when you are setting your habits, you want to choose behaviors that will help you see results over the journey of five years as a minimum, so make sure the advice you listen to holds up under scrutiny and isn't just a passing trend or fad that will go out of fashion in a few months.

Holiday Marketing

Every holiday celebration seems to involve food of some kind, and very little of it tends to be healthy. Marketing agencies have altered our eating habits around these events to suggest we break our good habits and eat more sugary and fatty foods. Be wary of what you are consuming on holidays and try not to let it interfere too much with maintaining your habits. Easter is usually celebrated with mass amounts of chocolate, but there is no reason why these foods must be involved in your holiday schedule. Christmas involves all kinds of unhealthy foods like heavily processed ham, cookies, pudding, and other desserts. Valentine's Day is all about chocolate, but some beautiful roses might make for a suitable substitute. Even sporting events are plagued by marketing for soft drinks, beer, hot dogs, and junk food.

You do not need to give these kinds of foods up entirely, but it does help to moderate how much of it you eat during a holiday. Do your best to stick to your healthy habits rather than falling into marketing pitfalls that encourage overindulgence and see where you can substitute healthy or non-food alternatives.

No Plan = No Direction

If you don't know what your end goal is and how you plan to get there, how can you begin to work towards it? A solid plan is imperative for success. If you want to get ahead, make a Personal Growth

Development Plan that includes all the outcomes you want to achieve and what you need to do to pull off those outcomes. Brian Tracy, bestselling author and top international speaker, says that Personal Growth Development Plans largely focus on the process of setting your goals, making a plan and schedule for reaching those goals, and concentrating on the high-value goals. He encourages people to take their time to decide on what they are trying to do before they start working so they know which direction to head. Whatever your big dream or goals are, keep them in your thoughts as you commit yourself to establish and to maintain better habits. Once you know what you are trying to do, you can start planning and organizing your daily habits to support the goals you wish to achieve.

Structuring Your Day

Scheduling your habits throughout the day can be the difference between diligently keeping them and letting them fall by the wayside. Think about what you want to accomplish each day. These should be small scale changes and activities that you can repeat and turn into habits over time. Then arrange these actions into a schedule that fits with your needs and your lifestyle, creating patterns and routines you stick to nearly every day.

Routines in the morning and evening are very important, so focus on these to begin with. Morning routines help you wake up refreshed and ready to succeed over all of the day's challenges. Routines in the morning and evening "prime you for success. They help you achieve more, think clearly, and do work that matters. They keep you from stumbling through your day and make sure you get the most important things done" (Altrogge, 2019, para. 3). Evening routines help you wind down from a busy day and get enough sleep for the next day. Structuring your day around habits and routines that support your health and fitness will help you get closer to your goals each day.

G.O.A.L.S
Goals Offer Alternative Life Stories

Goal setting establishes clarity on what you need to do to develop the right habits and therefore making adjustments to your subsequent behaviors that will build your momentum. Your goals will give you a measure of control over your life that you may not have had otherwise because it can direct you towards a target or purpose instead of leaving you to just drift through life. Once you know which direction you should be going, you can take the appropriate steps to get there.

Brian Tracy also says that goals help you take notice of your progress by giving you a metric to measure them against. If you are trying to get in shape, you may get discouraged if you don't feel you are making much progress, but after assessing the situation, you may realize that while you have not yet met your goal, you have made significant progress from where you began. Knowing your finish line lets you track your progress and see the impact your small changes have made. Goals allow you to create a new path and develop brand new opportunities, life experiences, and stories. They help you become aware of the actions you need to take every day to succeed. You only need to know how to use them to their full effect.

DR. ACTION™

DR. ACTION™ is a goal-setting strategy that I developed that will help you identify the outcomes that matter most to you and get the most out of your goals. It will help walk you through the process of determining your ideal outcome and strategizing how you want to go about achieving it. This system is described in more detail in my book *Magnetic Goals*, but here is a brief overview of each component.

- Dream Big - Dream big and stretch yourself. Get clarity on what you want.
- Relevant - Make it personal and relevant to you.
- Action - Take immediate action and write up your big goals.
- Coordinates - Develop your plan and course of action steps.
- Time - Develop concrete time frames that are realistic for your goals.
- Implement - Follow through with your commitment and start.
- Opportunity - Be observant of opportunities that will present themselves.
- Now - Begin your journey now - your dreams can become a reality.

Understanding and implementing the steps of this process will help you develop goals that inspire change.

Dream Big

The first stage of goal setting is using your imagination and visualization skills to think of the things you want to achieve. Picture your perfect future life and what that life involves. Be bold and think big, and don't get caught up in what seems realistic and what doesn't. These goals should be incredibly empowering when you think of them as achievable. They need to be able to drive you through the tough times and encourage you to push yourself, so they need to be things you have a strong attachment to that will help you remain resilient even when the road ahead seems tough.

Start by simply visualizing your future and thinking of everything you want to achieve. What would your perfect house be like, your ideal family vacation and your perfect lifestyle? What do your health and fitness goals need to be to get you there? What would your ideal fitness level look like? Once you have thought of these end goals, attach a reason or purpose to each one.

Relevant

Your goals should matter to you. Whether or not they live up to others' expectations is irrelevant. You are the one being motivated by the goals, so do not let the opinions of others get in the way of pursuing what you want. If your goals are deeply personal and meaningful, you will find it easier to develop a near-obsessive focus on achieving them rather than trying to push yourself to do something you don't have any real passion for. Think about what makes certain goals relevant to you and what differentiates them from those you have no passion for. What will this goal mean to you when you achieve it? What positive impact will it have on you and perhaps friends and family that will also benefit from it being achieved? You must know the answers to these questions when you set your goals.

Relevance is also important because you will be taking actions to achieve your goals every single day. There is no day off when you are working towards success, and even the rest days are meant to help you recuperate so you can be ready to get to work again the next day. If you are going to commit yourself to repeat an action every day for months or years, you need to care about what you are doing so you can keep putting energy into your actions. Take ownership of your goals, as they need to be yours and yours alone.

Action

Once you have established your goals, the next step is to start taking action. Nothing gets done unless you start doing it. There is no time for procrastination and hesitation. Start by writing down your goals so you can easily reference them to remind yourself what you are working for. Writing down your dreams is a bit like the process of inking a tattoo; you are laying out the groundwork upon which the color of the goal tattoo will be filled in. Your lines need to be strong, so they can guide your future endeavors.

The process of writing goals helps sow the seeds of development in your subconscious. It keeps the goals at the forefront of your mind and gives you some accountability for completing the goals because you have made a contract with yourself to finish them. From this, future growth will spring. If you neglect to write your goals and allow yourself to procrastinate starting on your goals, you cannot expect anything to change. If you want to see real, measurable differences in your health and fitness, you need to take action.

Coordinates

Just like on a real map, your coordinates show you where you currently are, and the coordinates of your destination show you where you need to go. They are the plan that will take you from one place to the other. If you start with a well-thought-out plan, you will not stumble as you proceed through the path to success.

Without a plan, you cannot know where you are headed, and so you will not know where you are going to end up. You could end up veering off course or, worse, completely stagnating and giving up on your goals. You want to avoid taking this risk, so make sure your plan contains actionable steps you can use to keep moving forward. Making a plan and establishing your coordinates means your mind will subconsciously begin to work through the steps and make choices that bring you closer to making your dreams become a reality.

Time

Great goals have time limits that are specific and realistic while still encouraging you to always keep making progress. Your mind will do a lot of the heavy lifting for you for this step, as it has a good idea of how long it will realistically take you to do something. Once set, the deadline will remain in the back of your mind, subconsciously pushing you to make sure you are getting everything done that you need to each day.

Once you have an overarching timeline, you can break down each step of your goal plan into its own time frame. Will a certain action take you a month, or is it something that you could reasonably get done in a week? Can you complete the first stage of your journey in a year? These questions help you set the pace of your journey and keep you on track for finishing on time.

Allocating a certain amount of time to each goal helps you prioritize the actions you need to take to achieve it. If you set no time limit on finishing reading a book, it may sit unread for months. If you tell yourself, you must finish it in three weeks; you are more likely to pick up the book every time your eyes pass over it. On many occasions, one goal's completion will lead right into the next. To keep on track, complete your 12-month goals so you can move closer to your two years goals, and so on.

Your time frame also gives you a good idea of the parameters you have and provides you with a sense of accountability for completing your goals on time. As you stay on track and draw closer to the deadline, you can prepare to celebrate your accomplishments.

Implement

The implementation phase is when all of your dreaming and planning comes to a head. Many people do not make it to the implementation phase. They spend all their time thinking about what their life could be like, but they never step up and put their goal plans into practice. If you want to achieve your goals, the magic begins here. Just starting to implement your plan lets you kickstart your motivation and gets you on track. If you can manage to take that first step and make the commitment to following through on your plans, you will have a huge chance of actually reaching your goals so long as you stay true to the course. Simply start your journey and follow the path you have made for yourself, and the rest will come easily to you.

Opportunity

Opportunities are always around us, and frequently we let them pass by without even noticing their presence. It is up to you to recognize them and take advantage of them when they appear. If you don't make the most out of your opportunities when they arise, they are often passed on to others, while you remain exactly where you began.

The opportunity component of DR. ACTION™ is all about awareness. Learn to recognize the signs of an opportunity so you can make the most of it. You can make this process easier by reviewing your goals regularly, which tunes your mind into things that will help you get ahead and accomplish your objectives. When an opportunity does arrive, take action. If you need to make a phone call, send an email, or get in touch with someone for a follow-up conversation, do so as soon as possible. Don't let the task sit around for a few days while you debate whether or not to do it. If you procrastinate on an amazing opportunity, you just might find that it is no longer available when you finally get around to it.

Now

The final step of the DR. ACTION™ process is to act now, not later. You've completed all the preliminary work you need to get to this point. It is the time to put all of your planning into action right now. Let your motivation and momentum carry you forward and get off on the right foot. You will need a significant personal commitment, clear daily structure, a good plan, courage, and the ability to tackle your hesitations with ruthless perseverance, but so long as you keep taking action, you can achieve your goals.

Chapter 3

STOP>REVIEW>PIVOT and POWER

Progress reports allow businesses to see how much work and improvement a person or team has made on a project. They are essential for ensuring deadlines are being met, and progress is being made. But what if you could use a progress report to review your situation in regards to your health and fitness? I designed the *STOP>REVIEW>PIVOT* and *POWER* system so that my clients have an opportunity to review and reflect on where they currently are and change direction if their current course is not taking them where they need to go. It also supplies its users with the power to build up their momentum and make a real impact on their lives. With this system, you can develop an honest assessment of your current status and understand what needs to be changed in order to achieve success.

The system is made up of four components, each of which has a unique purpose that helps you self-evaluate. The steps will help you identify if your current habits are progressing your chances to achieve a healthy lifestyle, or if your habits are hindering the opportunity to obtain a suitable balance of your fitness level and a healthy diet. By placing the habits you engage in every day under the microscope, you can get a good sense of what's working and what's holding you back that may otherwise have been left unnoticed.

Each step will be explained in more detail, but first, I want to give a brief explanation of what the steps of the system do.

The first step, **STOP**, asks you to pause and consider the exact moment you are in right now. Don't think about where you were a year ago, and don't count anything you plan on doing in the future. Just focus on the here and now and pinpoint if, at this very moment, your current daily habits are taking you in your intended direction.

Next, **REVIEW** requires you to look at your answer and identify what is working well and separate it from what isn't. What changes would you need to implement to get back on course? Can you identify any triggers that have a history of causing you to lapse in your determination and undo all the progress you have made so far and will make in the future?

PIVOT is the process of beginning to implement the changes you have identified during your review. This may be only a marginal change of direction or an increase in your commitment to your goals, or it may involve an entire overhaul of your plan and new goals you wish to achieve. In nearly all circumstances, you will still use the process of introducing mini habits to make these new changes. In the final stage, **POWER**, your renewed commitment and clarity will give you purpose. This provides you with the energy you need to push forward knowing you have conducted a thorough review, you have the right action plan in place, and you are now in the perfect position to achieve your fitness, diet, and overall health goals.

STOP - Where Do You Sit Right Now on a Scale of One to 10?

It can be a challenge to grade your current performance in relation to your goals to pinpoint precisely how you are tracking. To help you, I want to walk you through the actionable steps so you can conduct your very own performance review with the *STOP>REVIEW>PIVOT* and *POWER* system.

The first step is taking time to reflect and giving yourself a grade on your current position. You can fill out the questions as I guide you through the process, and this is all about taking *ACTION* in the moment. So, take out a notebook and a pen or pencil and answer the following questions with either of three options being yes, no, or occasionally. Your answers will provide you with just a basic level of your current condition, but you can refer back to them at any future point as they form a great reference point you can continue from.

Exercise/Fitness:

1. Do you exercise for a minimum of 30 minutes a day, five days per week?

2. When exercising, do you reach a point of perspiration in at least two of your sessions each week?

3. Do you have time in the day specifically set aside to exercise?

4. Do you find ways to make exercise fun and participate in activities you enjoy?

5. Do you always introduce new fitness habits incrementally into your schedule because you view these new habits from a long-term perspective?

6. Are you conscious of activities considered to be high impact and the risk associated with these activities on your joints as you age? For example, swimming, golf, yoga, and cycling are low impact activities. Basketball, netball,

hockey, and running on hard surfaces are considered high impact activities.

Diet/Nutrition:

1. Do you eat a minimum or the equivalent of two handfuls of fresh vegetables and two handfuls of fruit (if cut up into pieces) each day?

2. Do you drink a minimum of two litres of water each day?

3. Do you make a conscious effort to ensure that your breakfast does not contain high levels of fats, high levels of sugars, or more than a cup of dairy products like milk and cheese?

4. Do you understand that marketing can significantly influence you and condition you to eat the wrong foods, and therefore stay away from gimmick "diet fads"?

5. Are you committed to restricting too much snacking throughout the day, particularly with items full of sugar and preservatives?

6. Are you always health-conscious when doing your shopping and do you rotate your nutrition sources, so you are not eating the same foods day in and day out?

Now, add up your score based on your answers. Each *YES* is worth five points, each *OCCASIONALLY* is worth three points, and each **NO** is worth one point. Compare your total score to the following score summaries.

Summarizing your score

A combined score between **12 and 25** indicates there are numerous negative habits that will need to be addressed and adjusted across your diet and exercise patterns. Don't get disheartened; this is not about negative judgment. Instead, it is about self-reflection at this very moment and taking this fantastic opportunity to identify some simple but effective changes you can implement in the form of mini habits that will help you bring up your score. Importantly, you are absolutely on the right track, and I commend you for this. You have taken the right action by reading The Habit Switch, and you are ready to commit to a lifelong change. As you continue to read and implement your plan for improving your health and fitness, stop and take action when required. Start to implement healthy habits into your daily routine that will replace some of the less supportive ones you may still use.

A combined score of **26 to 45** suggests you have identified some areas of potential improvement. Adding a few extra mini habits to your schedule to bolster your current diet and exercise plans will help you further improve your score. You have a firm grasp on the basics of keeping yourself healthy, but there are still a few ways in which you can significantly improve your long-term health and well-being with additional incremental changes.

A combined score between **46 and 60** indicates that you are tracking very well across your health and fitness. You are likely engaging in mini habits already that help to keep your momentum moving towards your goals. Even if you score high on this preliminary questionnaire, you have likely noticed there are some areas you can continue to improve in. Remember, the above questions will provide a baseline feel for your current habits and that they do not represent all the things you could be doing to get and stay healthy. We will dive deeper into other areas of exercise and diet that will enable you to take your health and fitness to another level later in the book.

At this point, the initial step of **STOP** helps you identify some of the amazing benefits of a healthy lifestyle and where these benefits can come into play in your own life. These include:

- Improving your self-esteem and self-confidence
- Improving your clarity of mind, memory, and focus
- Reducing the risk of many diseases including cardiovascular disease, stroke, and diabetes
- Improving your flexibility, muscle strength, and range of movement
- Helping you maintain balance and coordination as you age
- Significantly reducing the onset of osteoporosis and lessening the chances of bone fractures
- Improving your ability and speed for recovering from various illnesses
- Reducing the symptoms of stress, anxiety, and depression, subsequently improving your sense of well-being and happiness

Stopping and making an assessment of where your current habits are steering you allows you to keep ahead of the pack on your fitness journey and get closer to achieving all of these benefits and more.

REVIEW - Reflection and Observation

A review of your plan needs to be an ongoing process that you regularly conduct so you can determine if you are moving in the right direction. You may require some course correction, and it can be helpful when you first commence to review yourself initially after one month, then three months, and then every six months after that. Part of this focus for reviewing your goals is to ensure you are preparing yourself adequately to achieve your desired outcomes, and also that you still want to pursue the goals you have chosen.

Start to think about the decisions that you have made up to this point. Which ones have benefitted your progress, and which ones have hindered it? Being able to review your past choices and current habits gives you insight into what is working and what isn't so that you can more effectively target the areas in need of improvement.

Reflection is helpful in many fields, not just fitness. It allows us to recognize our blind spots and fix them where we can. It is an opportunity for inward reflection, but not one for being overly critical of yourself. This is because you are currently in a transitionary period of change, and change takes time. It is unfair to expect yourself to be much farther than you are without giving yourself the proper time to enact the change you want to see. If your focus on your goals has slipped, think about why this may have happened and what you can do to get it back on track, not on berating yourself.

In goal setting, there is a lot of temptation always to look forward and never look back. You are focused on what you should do next and how it will help you achieve your goals. But taking the time to look backwards and evaluate your performance to date can be helpful too. You want to always keep your goals in mind, but you need to celebrate and appreciate what you have achieved on your journey. Past mistakes and successes both need to be acknowledged as they will assist in changing or reinforcing the decisions that initially led to them.

During the Review stage, make sure to always remain honest with yourself and remember that reflection is a wonderful learning opportunity. Your improvement may be impacted, and you will never be able to make the appropriate changes if you don't give yourself a genuine review. You do not need to be overly critical, but you should consider what you could have done differently in a given situation.

Only an honest view will show how you can improve.

An Example Review

If you are still a little unsure of what an effective review looks like, use the following example. You can adjust the questions to fit your own goals more specifically if needed.

My Health Review (conducted after one month):
Date:

1. The new supportive habits I have introduced since my last review are:
2. The habit(s) that I have had difficulty implementing since my previous review have been:
3. Out of 10, how would I honestly rate my current progress?   /10
4. If my rating is under 6/10, what will I need to do to lift my rating to an 8/10?
5. If I rated yourself higher than a 6/10, what habits would I need to implement to score 10/10?
6. Do I still feel that my clarity and focus are always aligned to my ideal desired outcomes?

7. What have been my biggest challenges or roadblocks since the previous review?

8. If I identified roadblocks or particular challenges with introducing my supportive mini habits, what do I need to do to 'pivot' and change direction?

9. What are the top five mini habit goals that I wish to achieve prior to my next review?

10. What is my plan to incrementally introduce these habits with a long-term view? That is, if these habits were to be part of my day for the next five years, how would I introduce the habit slowly, over a 60-90 day period?

The ability to give yourself an honest review is an invaluable skill, but not one that comes easily to everyone. If you need further guidance on the process, try making use of the following resources:

- *La Trobe University's (Australia)* "_Reflective Practice in Health_" *for a step-by-step guide to reflection*

- *The Telegraph's* "_Six Daily Decisions that can Make or Break Your Health_" *for more information about differentiating between good and bad decisions*

PIVOT - A Change of Direction

You know what's working and what's not. Now it's time to take that knowledge and implement it. There are two possible results from the Review process. The first is that you may find that you are on track to complete your goals and you do not have to make changes to your approach after all, or the changes you need to make are very minimal. In this case, proceed with the groundwork you have laid down, making the small adjustments and additions you have identified. With perseverance and time, you will reach your health and fitness goals. Don't attempt to tweak things if your only goal is speeding up the process. As we have discussed, real change takes time and trying to rush it can lead you to unfortunate side-effects.

The other possible result from the Review process is that you have identified a few or more areas that would benefit from alterations, additions, and replacements for negative habits that are impeding your progress. This result tends to be more common as we slip back into old behavior patterns and our focus wavers on our goals. It is nothing to be ashamed of, especially if you are just starting out on making serious improvements to your health. So long as you can rebound from it, this can actually be a result that helps reinvigorate you. It is always better to identify these less than helpful habits sooner rather than later. The good news is that now that you have identified the problem, you can take the proper steps to correct it.

Habit Pivoting

Pivoting your habits is the process of replacing negative habits with positive ones. If you have decided that a particular habit is no longer helping you reach your goals, swap it out for one that will. This can be as simple as increasing 20 minutes of daily exercise to 30 minutes, or it could mean something more involved, like starting a new exercise routine entirely.

If you need to make significant changes, make sure you are implementing them incrementally. Start with small intervals of exercise and dietary changes and slowly transition to new habits over time. Evaluate the direction of your new plan to decide how quickly new habits should be implemented and what your expected results will be.

Goal Pivoting

In some cases, you may find that your current goals no longer resonate with you, and you need to change your goals themselves. This can be a tough call to make, but if it is necessary, then you are better off pivoting than trying to pursue something you no longer feel passionate about. Taking steps to make a change happen when you notice one coming lets you decide the direction you will pivot and gives you agency. If you wait too long, often life has a way of making the change without your input and taking you along for the ride (Sreenivasan, 2017, para. 3). Take the opportunity to sit and write down your new desired outcomes so you can repeat the goal-setting process. When you have successfully shifted your goals, you can begin deciding on the new habit plan for achieving the outcomes you have chosen to pursue.

POWER - A Renewed and Committed Focus for Your Health

The final part of the system is to power onwards! All the revisions you have made to your plan should leave you feeling more committed than ever before. With the renewed energy and focus you are feeling, you can keep pushing forward and using your mini habits to your advantage.

Remember that your review process represents a commitment to yourself. If you have identified areas in need of change, you have to follow through and make those changes. Keep the daily reminders of your habits and goals easily visible, so you stick to them. Make yourself a well-structured schedule you can follow that keeps you accountable for completing all of your habits each day.

An ongoing investment in your health is critical for all other fields of self-improvement. You spend so much of your time trying to benefit others. Take some time to improve yourself and make sure your body is always running at peak performance. After all, you need a healthy, reliable body to carry you to achieve all of your goal. That is why you must take your new habits and goals seriously and fully commit yourself to them.

Completing a self-review every 3 – 6 months is a minimal time commitment. Set aside just one hour every three to six months so you can work through the review process, adjust the direction you are moving, and then power forward to achieve success.

Confidence Builders - The 1 % Changes

Momentum and change build confidence. We need to view our progress as motivational and let it carry us through to future successes. When you really care about what you are doing, every step you take will feel like its own success. These simple, one percent changes that you make every day or even every week can exponentially improve your self-esteem, especially when you learn to recognize their huge compounding impact.

Ongoing improvements always make a difference, no matter how small. If you cut candy out of your diet, even if it doesn't lead to immediate weight loss, you are still taking steps to make yourself healthier. If you expand on this change with a series of continuous improvements, you will find that in a year or two, you end up leagues ahead of where you began. It may seem unglamorous at first. We are bombarded by success stories of how people made millions overnight or lost 20 pounds in two weeks, and while these stories are alluring, they represent one in a million odds. The difference between them and your path to progress is that everyone can make a one percent change, repeated over time, without any need for luck. James Clear, author of

Atomic Habits says that it may be true that getting one percent better isn't going to make headlines but there is one thing about it, though: it works". You are using the tortoise method of "slow and steady" here, not the hare, which means you avoid risks like burnout. The one percent changes you make will boost your confidence and take you ever closer to your goal.

Making a 1% Change Every Day

One percent does not seem like a lot on its own, but just like habits, it can build up into something amazing. You only need to be willing to commit yourself to make tiny improvements regularly. To become one percent better each day, you need to focus on your reasons for self-improvement, the personal gratification you feel when you improve, maintaining a long-term view, and ensuring you take action consistently. Taking action is the most crucial step because without action, you will never achieve your outcomes.

If you were to change just one thing about yourself or your actions each day, do you know how much you could achieve over time? To show the amazing change you can achieve, take the example of money.

If you were to start with just $100 at the beginning of the year and you were able to increase what you have by 1% every single day, at the end of the year, you would have accumulated $3,778.34 [or] 37.7 being 8x what you had at the beginning of the year. We are used to seeing compound gains like this when it comes to money, but personal improvement works the same way. One improvement will lead to the next, and before long, you will be just so far ahead of where you once were. Even if you were to make a one percent improvement every day for 100 days, only ⅓ of a year, you would be 100% better than you were when you started. The small improvements matter as long as you keep the ball rolling and remember to take smart, beneficial actions each day.

Chapter 4

How to Switch on Your Diet Habits

You can make significant improvements to your health through your diet using the mini habit method. Small changes in what you eat and how you approach eating will help you regain control over your eating habits. Learning how to flip on the habit switch and improve your diet is a matter of altering your mindset. If you want to eat healthily, lose weight, and continue to eat foods that give you energy rather than make you lethargic and exhausted, you must break free of the constraints of your old habits and be prepared to change the way you think about dieting and the power of different food sources.

Are You Prepared to Switch? - How to Turn off Your Former Diet Habits

We all have a set of dietary habits that determine our approach to our nutrition. The formation of these habits can be attributed to a few different factors, many of which begin in our childhood. If you ate and were told of the great benefits of eating vegetables as a child, you are more likely to have developed a taste and an appreciation for vegetables as an adult. The opposite is also true; if you had to be convinced to finish a side of broccoli as a child, you have likely built up negative associations that get in the way of eating healthy food as an adult. In this way, our dietary habits have a massive impact as we grow from children to teenagers to adults and get to choose our meals. Some negative dietary habits, usually those that are developed later in life, are often easy to recognize and change. Those that we have carried with us since childhood, almost appear to be ingrained in our subconscious mind, making them very difficult to change.

As children, we make negative and positive associations toward all kinds of food. If you were 'forced' to eat a particular type of food that you did not enjoy, you likely resented that food and hated seeing it on your plate. It can be just small things as a child that can become the stimulus that can cause negative habits later in life.

The only way to change these habits is to change the way you approach your meals, first by recognizing the power of past and current eating habits on future ones. Remove the mindset that you can, or your children can eat what you or they want while young because positive and supportive habits begin early and you establish the right foundations that will take you through at a very early age.

If for example, you spend your 20's eating bacon "while apparently you still can," you will likely continue to eat bacon well into your 40's and 50's, when the compounding impact of cholesterol can cause heart and other cardiovascular diseases. If you always think "I'll worry about that later" in regards to eating habits, when "later" finally comes those habits will be so ingrained that they will be difficult to shake.

Everything circles back to your goals and desired outcomes. What do you want to accomplish, and what would you like to avoid? This also applies to present-day health concerns you may be currently facing, not just future ones. Maybe cardio-vascular disease runs in your family, and you are looking to buck the trend. Perhaps you have young children, and you want to have enough energy to share activities with them without being out of breath. Whatever your current and future health goals are, they matter to you, so you must be willing to embrace change and break free from old habits to achieve them.

Most importantly, you have already taken your first step towards leading a healthy and uncomplicated life by picking up this book as mentioned in the introductory. I am a firm believer that certain books have come into my life at just the right times when I needed to hear their message the most. If this is true for you too, then you know that you must take the step that 90% of the population fails to do and take action, now, to implement the suggestions outlined here. Remember, The Habit Switch is all about simplicity, maintaining common sense, and practical diet habits that are sustainable in the long term. I strongly encourage you to make use of the ideas that work best for you and stick to your plan. If this is your first book about habit change for your diet, make it your last for a minimum of 12 months. If at the end of that period you find that the suggestions are not sustainable then yes, look for alternatives, but really, give these ideas time to grow first.

I want to help you by breaking information down by simplifying the steps as much as possible. My background as a teacher has provided me with the ability to break information down into smaller and more manageable steps that have been a proven method for success. Make your personal promise to 'switch' your current habits into those that will significantly improve your health for the long term.

Why a switch can add years to your life

Sticking to healthy habits will allow you to spend more time doing the activities you enjoy. In fact, some healthy habits can even add years onto your lifespan, giving you incredible amounts of extra time to get more done. A recent Harvard University study found that you can increase your life expectancy by over a decade if you follow certain healthy habits. The five habits identified in the study are:

1. not smoking;
2. having a body mass index between 18.5 and 25;
3. taking at least 30 minutes of moderate exercise a day;
4. having no more than one 150 mL glass of wine a day for women, or two for men. Personally, I think water is best anyway!
5. Having a diet rich in items such as fruit, vegetables and whole grains and low in red meat, saturated fats and sugar.

(Harvard University, 2018, para. 7)

These small changes build up into a tremendous impact on your overall health.

Most of the habits in the study are common sense suggestions, and many are relatively easy to implement in to your life style. The power of "mini things" is readily apparent here. It does not take a lot to have a big impact on your fitness; it only takes many small things combined over time.

Regarding the consumption of no more than 150 mL of alcohol each day, I suggest limiting alcohol whenever possible. The problem for alcohol with many people is that it encourages snacking on cheese, crackers, or other high-fat food while they drink. This introduces unnecessary excess calories that could be avoided just by avoiding alcohol as often as you can.

Sustainable Diets are not Complicated!

In this section, I want to turn what may at times, feel complicated and overwhelming into easy to process information. I believe an effective diet must be easily understandable so that you know what you should be doing, and you have everything you need to succeed. Back when I was in school, I found some classes challenging because of the way the material was taught. It was assumed I knew certain prerequisite information, but this was incorrect.

Some teachers tended to assume I was learning what was being taught, but I was missing important information and had to work twice as hard to catch-up. This is precisely what I want to avoid with my own teaching style as I walk you through developing your healthy habit plan. You should be able to have a firm grasp on the information being presented to you without risk of complex topics that leave you behind, so I have simplified my lesson plan. Get ready for a fast-track lesson on how to make a change to a healthy diet uncomplicated!

There are many different diets that are currently popular. I do not believe there is much value in comparing the pros and cons of each, as I want to focus more on giving you a brief overview of these diets. This is so you can see just how confusing it is for people without a background in anatomy, physiology, and nutrition to determine what is suitable and useful and what is just plain ludicrous. I do have my personal opinions about each of these diets, but as you continue to read about my belief systems for leading a healthy life through diet and exercise and the right foods to be eating, you can start to see where some of these trendy diets falter, especially when viewed as potential long-term solutions. Again, I'm not here to criticize and dissect the various diets that are available, instead show you how there can be contradictory diet information just across these 6 current popular diets.

The Paleo Diet

The paleo diet, as the name suggests, encourages people to eat in a way similar to their ancestors. This means cutting out processed foods, sugar, and grains. Essentially, you limit your diet to veggies, meat, fruit and nuts. Underpinning these dietary restrictions is the theory that the modern Western diet, full of dairy, grains, and processed foods, is responsible for the high rates of many diseases. Paleo tries to cut down on the number of carbohydrates in your diet in an attempt to keep these diseases at bay and encourage weight loss. According to the diet, "the fewer number of carbohydrates in your system leads to a decreased amount of glucose. So your system will then begin to use fat as its fuel source" (NutritionED, n.d., para. 2). Theoretically, by restricting carbs, you encourage your body to burn fat instead.

Plant-based or vegan diet

The vegan diet and other plant-based diets limit the foods in the diet to only those that come from plants, such as fruits, vegetables, legumes, and plant-based meat and dairy alternatives. It is an extension of the vegetarian diet that excludes animal products as well as meat. Proponents of using veganism for weight loss say it works "because its very low fat and high fiber content may make you feel fuller for longer" (Bjarnadottir, 2019, para. 3). This is an opposite approach to many low-carb diets, which typically have higher fats, lower fiber, and almost always include meat products. Many people engage in plant-based diets for moral reasons rather than purely weight loss ones, though some dieters have simply chosen to eat animal product-free because they believe in the health benefits.

The Atkins Diet
The Atkins diet is a type of low-carb diet that emphasizes both proteins and fats, which it suggests are meant to keep your fuller for longer periods of time. Proponents of the diet "insist that you can lose weight by eating as much protein and fat as you like, as long as you avoid carbs"

(Bjarnadottir, 2019, para. 7). Its main goal is weight loss. The diet is split into four phases, each of which has different requirements for how much of your diet is made up of carbs, proteins, and fat. The Atkins diet also claims that "obesity and related health problems, such as type 2 diabetes and heart disease, are the fault of the typical low-fat, high-carbohydrate American diet" (Mayo Clinic Staff, 2017, para. 6). People who follow the diet increase their fat intake rather than cutting down on it, and instead focus on limiting carbs.

Intermittent Fasting

Intermittent fasting is a process of eating during certain hours and fasting during others. It does not suggest avoiding any particular types of food; instead, it provides guidelines for when you should be eating. There are many different eating patterns involved in intermittent fasting, each one suggesting different intervals of time between meals and sometimes different times of day when it is more optimal to fast or eat. By nature, it requires you to skip meals throughout the day. Sometimes this can become more extreme periods of time, as "common intermittent fasting methods involve daily 16-hour fasts or fasting for 24 hours, twice per week" (Gunnars, 2018, para. 2). The fasting is meant to reduce your overall caloric intake, which in turn leads to weight loss.

The Keto Diet

The keto diet is a more extreme version of low-carb diets like Atkins. It suggests eliminating nearly all carbohydrates from your diet and supplementing them with higher fat intake. This effectively removes an entire macronutrient from your meals. Supporters of the diet say it "lowers blood sugar and insulin levels, and shifts the body's metabolism away from carbs and towards fat and ketones," which act as alternative energy sources (Mawer, 2018, para. 3). A successful keto diet attempt involves entering a state known as ketosis, where your body shifts to these alternative fuels and burns stored fat. Keto diet plans are full of high-fat foods like red meat, nuts, eggs, and even the fairly frequent incorporation of bacon, which is typically viewed as a cause of weight gain, not the solution to it.

The TLC Diet

The TLC diet does not stand for tender loving care, as the typical use of the acronym would have you believe. Instead, it is short for Therapeutic Lifestyle Changes. It suggests making food selections that benefit your heart health. Typical distribution of nutrients on the diet encourages dieters to get "50-60% of their daily calories from carbs, 24-35% from fat, and 15% from protein" (Sass, 2019, para. 2). The TLC standard diet includes plenty of vegetables, fruit, whole grains, nuts, and low fat or nonfat dairy. It also allows for low-fat protein selections like fish and skin-off poultry. It is designed primarily for keeping cholesterol low, though it is believed to have weight loss benefits as well.

Eating for sustainability

Now that you have a brief background on these six dieting styles, let me outline what an easy and sustainable diet should consist of. We will delve into a few different areas, but my aim is to keep things simplified. Remember, there is no miraculous fix, no silver bullet that will let you shed dozens of pounds in no time without some hidden drawback. Your health is predominantly determined by ensuring you have a high intake of the right foods and nutrients rather than eliminating the bad foods in your diet. If you focus on eating the right food sources, you won't have to worry about eating the wrong things. Your nutritional needs need to be met in the most simplified, functional, and practical way possible. Before starting on any diet, ask yourself, is this diet sustainable for 10 years? If not, you may want to reconsider if it will help you achieve your long-term health goals.

The Eight Tips to Develop a Long-Term Healthy Habit Plan for Your Diet

Note that my intention in this section is not to dive deep into the specifics and design a healthy meal chart for breakfast, lunch, and dinner, nor am I giving you specific recipes you must follow with no wiggle room. Your meal plan needs are unique to you as an individual, and this level of meal planning may require the aid of a dietician or nutritionist to assist you over the course of several sessions. My aim is to provide a guideline, dispel some confusion, bring things into clear focus, and allow you to make healthy choices moving forward that you can implement with mini habits. This is the goal of my eight key tips to mastering healthy diet habits.

Healthy Tip 1
Mix it up!

All the different kinds of food we eat have different types and combinations of nutrients, vitamins, and minerals. There is no one food or tablet supplement that can supply us with all the nutrients we need to live a full and happy life, and your diet should reflect this. For example, bananas are high in vitamin C, vitamin B, and potassium, but they contain no vitamin E or magnesium. Almonds provide us with vitamin E and magnesium but no vitamin C or potassium. To fulfill all of your body's needs, you need to incorporate many different foods into your meals. Variety is imperative in any diet, and not just for health reasons. Eating a wide variety of foods helps you put more care into what you are eating and mix up your diet, which can lead you to try foods you've never had before and discover a new love for something you wouldn't have otherwise tried. Eating the same foods every week makes mealtime boring and makes it easy to stop paying attention to what you are putting in your body, especially if every week you are eating something that is not so healthy for you.

I would suggest you try adjusting your eating habits based on the current season, selecting produce that is at its freshest and making meals that compliment them. This means eating foods like watermelon, cucumbers, avocado, tomatoes, and other hydrating produce in summer, while winter diets are composed of foods such as stews, grains, nuts, carrots beans etc. You may already naturally be pulled towards these types of meals as the seasons change. Eating based on what is in season is a great way to create variety in your diet with the added benefit that they may be cheaper as they are in more abundance at that time of the year. Currently, most produce is available seasonally due to grocery stores' ability to stock foods from other parts of the world and store them for longer periods, but trying to pick up some locally grown produce at a local fruit and veg store.

Healthy Tip 2
Hydration

We all need water. But are you getting as much of it as you should be? Drinking enough water can help you cut down on how much you are eating and promote healthier eating habits and hydration. Drinking more water leaves less room for craving sugary drinks like soda and sweetened juices. Water is a natural source of hydration for your body, and it helps in so many ways. There is a reason you can only survive for a few days without any water because every cell, tissue, and organ in your body needs water to function at peak efficiency and if you are dehydrated, this can interfere with your body's ability to function. If you need help drinking more water, keeping a bottle of water nearby to encourage you to take a sip more often. You can add a slice of lemon or lime to mix up the flavor if you get tired of plain water. Small adjustments like these can go a long way in increasing how much water you drink each day.

Healthy Tip 3
Fiber is the natural chimney sweep!

Fiber helps your body function as it should. It keeps your digestive system regular, and a healthy supply of it prevents a variety of health problems from occurring. Fiber is found only in plant foods such as whole-grain cereals and breads, beans, peas, and many other fruits and vegetables. These plants have different types of fiber, so it is important to eat many different kinds so that your body has access to everything it needs for regular bowel function, reduced symptoms of chronic constipation, and potentially lower the risk for heart diseases and some cancers.

A good supply of fiber also helps the bacteria in your gut function properly. Bacteria is typically seen as a bad thing, but the bacteria that reside in your stomach are 'good' bacteria, the same kind that are targeted by probiotics and, as it turns out, high fiber diets. Your gut bacteria "are crucial for various aspects of your health, including weight, blood sugar control, immune function and even brain function" (Gunnars, 2018, para. 20). These bacteria can break down and thrive off the fiber in your diet, so make sure you are eating plenty to keep these functions in top shape.

Healthy Tip 4
Some Fats Can Clog Up Your Pipes

Despite the recent popularity of fats in certain diets, there are still many fats you should limit in your diet. Not all fats are equal, and from my experience and education, some are worse for your body than others. Fats and oils are in many snacks that we might not otherwise think of as fatty, like buttery crackers and anything fried. Some foods and food groups contain higher fats than others. Many foods in the dietary protein group, which contains meat, fish, poultry, eggs, beans, and nuts, are high in fats. However, this does not mean you must cut out all protein from your diet. Knowing the difference between the types of fats will help you make smart protein choices. To keep things as simple as possible, here is a brief breakdown of the different fats and what role they should play in your diet.

Saturated fats should be limited. They are primarily found in foods like red meat and milk products, as well as anything made with these products. The main concern with eating saturated fat is the buildup of cholesterol in your body. Your liver contains cholesterol receptors that break cholesterol down, but "eating too much saturated fat stops the receptors from working so well, so cholesterol builds up in the blood" (Heart UK, n.d., para. 6). This can lead to health conditions like a heart attack or stroke if not properly moderated. If you are looking to decrease saturated fats in your diet, you should pay careful attention to the fats section of ingredient labels. You can also choose lean meats like chicken, turkey, and fish instead of red meat for most of your meals. Making smart choices about how often you eat saturated fats can save you trouble in the long run.

Monounsaturated and *polyunsaturated* fats are generally seen as the less harmful counterparts to saturated fats. Monounsaturated fats are often found in things like olive oil and canola oil, while most other vegetable oils, nuts, and high-fat fish are good sources of polyunsaturated fat. While all fat should only be consumed in moderation, "eating moderate amounts of polyunsaturated (and monounsaturated) fat in place of saturated and trans fats can benefit your health" (A.D.A.M., 2018, para. 2). You need some fat in your diet, so it is best to stick to the healthier varieties.

Fats, despite their potential negative impacts, play a beneficial role in the body as well. They supply energy and essential fatty acids your body needs to function. They also help your body absorb fat-soluble vitamins A, D, E, and K. I suggest that rather than adopting a low-fat diet or aiming for no fat at all, it is important to focus on eating those beneficial 'good' fats like polyunsaturated fats and limiting harmful saturated fats. However, many people continue to have a diet high in saturated fat mainly due to a lack of knowledge in the food science area, the perceived cost of cheap takeout compared to cooking at home, and convenience. Knowing how to choose healthier fats will help you lead a healthier life.

Healthy Tip 5
Maintaining a Healthy Weight

People of all ages need to be a healthy weight. Our fitness levels are a product of the choices we make, which means that with the right choices, it is entirely possible to maintain a healthy weight. Many people use body mass index (BMI) to see if their weight is healthy for their size, but remember that your ideal weight can depend on several factors, including your height, age and sex. People who are overweight increase their risk for health conditions like high blood pressure, heart disease, diabetes, and breathing problems. Maintaining a healthy weight also means not undereating or dieting excessively either, as you need good nutrition and the energy from eating enough calories to keep yourself active and healthy.

Weight loss is greatly benefitted by physical activity along with a combination of consuming the right food in your diet. Aerobic exercises, such as walking, running, swimming, skipping, and playing high-intensity sports like soccer or basketball all help burn fat and calories. Staying active is an important part of any weight loss routine.

Healthy Tip 6
Consume Plenty of Vegetables, Fruits, and Grains

Fruits, vegetables, and grain products are key parts of a balanced diet. They provide important vitamins, minerals, complex carbohydrates in the form of starch and dietary fiber, and other substances that are necessary for a healthy life. They are also typically naturally low in fat, so long as they are prepared, cooked and served without too many additions.

I would encourage you to eat as many vegetables as you desire. Avoid deep-frying them or using additives like oils, sauces, or cheeses, but so long as you are sticking primarily to vegetables you can, for the most part, eat as you please.

When eating grains, be sure to choose healthier

varieties like whole wheat and ancient grains. White bread and other products made with refined white flour can have added sugars that get in the way of the benefits of whole grains.

Healthy Tip 7
Avoid Consuming Too Much Sugar and Salt

You likely already know to avoid added sugars and sweeteners, but too much sugar from natural sources can be a problem too. Sugars and starches occur naturally in foods that are otherwise nutrient-rich, including fruits, some vegetables, milk, beans, breads, cereals, and other grains. Sugars are simple carbohydrates, while other dietary carbs like starch and fiber are complex carbohydrates. During digestion, all carbs except fiber break down into sugars, which means the body cannot tell the difference between added sugars and those that occur naturally. As a result, you should be wary of the amount of sugar you are eating, even from natural sources like fruits and grains. Sugars should be used in moderation by most healthy people and only sparingly by those with low-calorie needs.

Sodium chloride, or salt, also occurs naturally in foods as well as being an additive. Whether you are eating foods already high in salt or seasoning your meals with a pinch of table salt, keep an eye on how much sodium you are consuming. Of course, salt is not all bad. In the body, it plays an essential role in the regulation of fluids and blood pressure. But too much of it can lead to health concerns. People at risk of high blood pressure can lower their risk by limiting the amount of salt they eat, so get rid of the salt and pepper shakers!

Healthy Tip 8
Choose a Low Cholesterol Diet

Your body is capable of producing the cholesterol it needs. Cholesterol can also be obtained through dietary sources, typically animal products. These include egg yolks, meat and organ meats like liver especially, fish, poultry, and milk products that can be high in fat. Choosing foods with less cholesterol will help you keep your blood pressure and blood cholesterol at healthy levels.

A side note for vegetarian diets....

Many people across the world eat vegetarian diets as a result of their culture, beliefs, or individual health needs. Some vegetarians eat milk products and eggs, and as a whole, they are still able to enjoy excellent health without meat in their diet. You can get enough protein on a vegetarian diet so long as the variety and amount of protein-heavy meat alternatives consumed are adequate. If you pursue a vegetarian diet, there are still quite a few sources of protein available to you. These include eggs and dairy, as well as other non-animal products like nuts, peanut butter, legumes, soymilk, and tofu (American Academy of Family Physicians, 2019, para. 10). Still, meat, fish and poultry are major contributors of iron, zinc, and vitamin B in most diets, so vegetarians should pay special attention to getting these nutrients from sources compliant with their dieting habits.

As previously mentioned, vegan diets are plant-based and contain no animal products. Because of this, it can be trickier to ensure your body is getting all of the necessary nutrients. One compound to keep in mind is vitamin B12 because it only comes from animal products. This vitamin is essential for the production of red blood cells as it does help to maintain healthy nerves and a healthy brain. Vegans must supplement their diets with other sources of B12. Additionally, vegan diets, particularly for children, require additional sources of vitamin D and calcium, which most people get from milk products.

High-quality input = High-quality output

What you put into your body defines what you get out of it. The food you eat provides the energy and nutrients that help your body function optimally and make sure you are always at your best. Nutrients from our diets also act as the building blocks of cell repair and injury prevention. Eating the right foods can help you in so many ways as they help boost your energy level, assist with protecting against some cancers, aide in concentration and make you feel happier and become more resilient to stress. The foods we choose to eat now will have long-term consequences on our health as we age. It is up to you to decide whether those consequences will be positive or negative. Again, we see the compounding impact of small behaviors over an extended period. If you make sure to eat well every day, you will see amazing returns on health, weight loss, and energy levels.

Practical Steps to Implement Your Habit Switch

Now that we have covered many areas of healthy food sources, it is time to look at the practical steps to implement the suggestions into your daily life. As we have already discussed, the basis of your new healthy change must come from small habits built incrementally into your life. This will lead to your behaviors changing when the new habits become automatic and replace any pre-existing negative habits. Just as weight gain can be a product of small changes, so too can weight loss.

We will begin our practical steps for a habit switch with the very basics and continue to build from there.

Practical Step 1

The 72-hour test and trial

Sit down and think carefully about which dietary goals you can achieve within three days from now. Why just three days? We want to initially focus on the small changes we can implement and review in

72 hours so you can know if they are effective. We will move on to setting longer-term goals later, but first, just focus on the small steps, not the lifetime benefits you will see if you keep taking them. Get some initial wins on the board, build your foundation for change, and encourage confidence.

As a reminder, building habits incrementally requires the following key elements:

1. Changes must be small and incremental with a long-term mindset.
2. You must have a compelling reason why habit change is necessary for you. What aspect of the change makes you excited to try it out?
3. Develop your plan for success.
4. Make the path ahead easy, with the least amount of resistance possible for yourself.
5. You must introduce a cue or reminder to complete the habit, such as a to-do checklist.

To help you out, here is an example of how the implementation phase might go. It is a three-step process made firstly by identifying the goal, establishing a reason why it matters, and then creating a plan to implement the change that will bring you to your goal.

- *Identification Stage*: I have identified that I need to drink 2,000 mL (approx. 4 – 5 large glasses) of fresh water per day and eliminate my soft drink consumption in the process.
- *My Why*: I know that soft drinks are very high in sugar and provide no health benefits, only empty calories. They can contribute to poor oral health and weight gain.
- *Three Day Implementation Plan*: Drink 500 mL of fresh water each day and reduce my soft drink consumption to no more than 330 mL (1 can of soft-drink) per day.

You will note that the three-day implementation plan does not yet meet the goal identified in the example. It is only a starting point you can continue to expand upon until your goal is being met or even exceeded. Now that you have your basic idea, you can begin to take action to implement it in your life. Again, start small and build your actions in tiny steps.

1. Plan on a Sunday

This is more personal preference than a hard and fast rule, but I find that it helps to make my plans on a Sunday. I like to start my week on Monday with the plans fresh in my mind, ready to make a change for the new week. Additionally, since Sunday is my rest day from physical activity, I have more time to plan and make adjustments if they are needed. If you have had little luck implementing plans before, I would suggest giving this a try.

2. Write up your 72-hour "Switch Plan."

Your Switch Plan should involve pinpointing two specific habits. First, isolate just one habit that you know will improve your overall health in the long term. Try to make your choice very specific and achievable. For example, take the previous scenario, where the positive habit is drinking 500 mL per water a day as a target. Next, identify a diet habit that you know has been detrimental to your health, preferably one that is related to the positive habit you want to introduce. Choose something that occurs relatively frequently for you. In this case, we will again use consuming soft drinks.

Now determine the incremental change that you can do over the next three days. This is not a lot of time, so think small. You may not be able to cut out soft drink entirely during this time, but you can probably cut it back to 330 mL a day if you tried. Likewise, you may not hit 2,000 mL of water in the first three days, but you could try to drink 500 mL or just three cups. You are trying to gradually reduce the bad habit by gradually increasing the good habit.

3. Make it easy

For the most part, your goals themselves are going to be easy. This is part of keeping them sustainable. The most challenging part is not doing the action itself, but remembering to do it and keeping up with it throughout the day. Drinking water is not hard, but it can slip your mind easily. To remedy this issue, find ways to remind yourself of your goals periodically. Here are a few sample methods for keeping drinking enough water at the forefront of your mind.

If you are trying to drink 500 mL of water, purchase and use a 500 mL water bottle. This way, you know exactly what that much water looks like and how close you are to completing your goal at any given time. You can easily track your progress just by looking at your water bottle. In time, you can build up to a larger 2L bottle, but for now, focus on the 72-hour goal. Also, try to resist the temptation of drinking the whole bottle in one go and getting it out of the way. We are trying to build a habit that eventually gets expanded to 2,000 mL, and it would be highly unusual to drink that much water at once and on a regular basis. Splitting up your hydration throughout the day encourages you to build the habit following the same schedule, so stick to 100-150 mL each time you drink and quench your thirst over a longer period. This will have the added benefit of reducing the urge for other drinks later in the day, as you still have water to drink.

This one may be obvious, but it is often overlooked. Keep the bottle nearby and place it somewhere you look at frequently throughout the day. Keeping it in your line of sight and easily accessible makes it easier to return to it throughout the day. This might mean keeping it on your office desk or taking it with you to place in the cupholder in your car. The added visual cue may be enough for you to take frequent sips throughout the day, but if not, set the alarm on your phone to go off in two-hour intervals reminding you to drink. Some water bottles even come equipped with built-in timers that flash to remind you to drink. These timers become a cue that "triggers your brain to initiate a behavior. It is a bit of information that predicts a reward" (Clear, n.d.-b, para. 11), in this case, better hydration. Think of it like conditioning yourself to anticipate drinking water and automate the process. Daily habits are best ingrained into our lives when we do an action frequently and not just every few days or once or twice a week, so be sure to stick to the timers you have set for the remainder of the 72 hours.

Practical Step 2

Increase the frequency

The 72-hour trial run is meant to ease you into a new habit. Now you can begin to increase the frequency that you perform the habit. Reflect on how the last three days went. Is there anything you need to tweak? Is the cue you have chosen to prompt the habit strong enough? Did you stick to the mini habits? Was it too hard, or too easy? Make any adjustments you need before proceeding. We are aiming to automate this behavior, so the more you perform it, and the more structured your behaviors are the greater success you will have in maintaining the habit.

At this point, you can use the *STOP>REVIEW>PIVOT* and *POWER* method to ensure the habit you have chosen is right for you and your incremental introduction is starting to make changes. Once you have reviewed, gradually increase the length of time you do the habit and the frequency of the habit each day. For example, if you now find it easy to drink 500 mL of water a day, you can move up to a 750 mL water bottle and aim to finish it daily for the next 14 days. Don't try to push too hard too fast; just focus on slow, incremental steps.

Practical Step 3

Structure

Give yourself the structure you need to succeed. I have personally found that if I write down the habit, I want to complete in my schedule and give myself the opportunity and motivation to do it during the day, I am about 80% more likely not just to do the habit but automate it. Grab a piece of paper and write your new habit down along with others as you introduce them. The physical process of writing down your goals is compelling, as it is a proven method for significantly multiplying your chances of success.

Let's look at a few examples of what giving your habits structure would look like.

- ***Introduction of Habit #1***: Writing down my top three priorities and key actions for the following day

- **Reason**: Introducing this habit would allow me to have clarity and focus on my most important tasks for the next day. I could go to bed confident in the progress I will make tomorrow, and I will allow my subconscious to arrange the next day while I sleep. I then have confidence that I can wake up ready to tackle my most important tasks.

- **Incremental Change**: I started by setting the alarm at 5:30 PM. Even if I hadn't finished my other work by then, I stopped and grabbed my notepad to write down just my number one priority for the next day. I did this for three days, after which I reviewed and increased this to two priorities for seven days. Again, I reviewed and then increased to three key tasks. I always listed my number one priority at the top and used tick boxes to mark my progress to build confidence.

- **Long-term Results**: From just this one successfully implemented habit, I found that I had much more clarity going into the next day. I was more relaxed at night, and my focus was crystal clear. Due to its success, I decided to create *The Daily Goal Tracker* resource that lets you track over 1,000 actions each year.

I found amazing success through a simple habit I could accomplish in just a few minutes of my time every day. When I expanded the initial single priority into two and then three priorities, my successes increased exponentially. Now take a look at this second example based around improving your diet.

- ***Introduction of Habit #2***: Eat fresh salmon twice per week.

- ***Reason***: Salmon is an incredible source of nutrients for your diet. It is a powerhouse food source that provides several impressive health benefits. The Omega-3 fatty acids alone have been linked to "decreasing inflammation, lowering blood pressure, reducing the risk of cancer and improving the function of the cells that line your arteries" (Spritzler, 2016, para. 8). It is also full of B vitamins, potassium, and antioxidants.

- ***Incremental Change***: Fresh salmon inherently requires you to eat it before it goes bad, which is why I prefer fresh to frozen, which can sit in the freezer for weeks or months and does not help you form a habit. Instead, buy fresh salmon and place it so it is directly in your line of sight every time you open the fridge, such as right on the top shelf. Start with about four weeks of having one serving of salmon over a week, review, and then increase the amount to two fillets a week.

- ***Important Note***: I am very aware of the high cost of salmon. Many people will say they cannot afford to purchase fresh salmon. But when all the benefits are considered, salmon is definitely worth the price tag. In fact, I would argue that you actually cannot afford not to eat it!

Practical Step 4
Be proud at the check-out!

When I go to the grocery store, I find it intriguing to look at what others are buying. What you place on the check-out counter is a direct reflection of your diet and the energy levels you will have for the week. If you make healthy choices, you will be proud to put your food selection on display.

Recently, as I was checking out at the grocery store, I noticed the purchases of a gentleman to my left in his late 50's. I took a peek and noticed he had laid out:

1. A large bag with 24 Chinese dumplings

2. Two large chocolate blocks, 500g each
3. A small bag with eight frozen fish cakes
4. A pack of four cinnamon donuts
5. Two bottles of cola
6. Pasta sauce
7. Two loaves of white bread

At even just a quick glance, you can tell this is not a healthy or sustainable diet. It may be a cheap and easy one, but when you start to make healthy purchases, you will feel the difference when you layout purchases you can be proud of. It is also a great way to review what you eat in a typical week. When you next head to the store, really take notice of the carts of those around you. Would you be proud to load up with processed and heavily packaged foods, or would you be happier knowing you have made the right choice for yourself? Your goal should be at least 50% of your cart being foods that are not prepackaged. These foods are generally unhealthy and often come packed with preservatives. They are more for the temporary enjoyment your brain gets from eating something sweet or salty, but ultimately unhealthy for your body's long-term benefit.

You should feel good about what you are eating. If

your guilty pleasure foods really make you feel guilty, consider why that is and if it is time to say goodbye to these guilty snacks. Make it a personal game to try to impress the people at the check-out and behind you in the line, and you will find it much easier to pick up fresh ingredients.

Practical Step 5
Organization and Application

Maintaining a healthy diet takes discipline and commitment. Your initial excitement and motivation may fade away over time when you get cravings for things you have left behind. Having the personal courage to continue making smart diet decisions, supported by good organization and planning, will keep you going. Having a clear goal and knowing the reason why you are doing all of this will help bolster your self-discipline. To accurately organize your healthy habits and apply them, you must take the proper steps to support your personal commitment.

This final practical step is inspired by the old-fashioned food pyramid that we may all have seen when you were a child. You will likely remember posters of this pyramid, maybe back in your grade school days, that provides a visual representation of what you should be eating and in what relative amounts. If you find that you sometimes slip into bad eating habits due to temptation in the fridge or pantry, try this instead.

Use your fridge and pantry to create a sort of visual food pyramid of your own, dividing up what you need to eat most and least of. The top shelf, the most readily available to your eye line when you open the fridge, should contain what you should eat most of. This includes foods like salmon, fresh vegetables, fruit, and other dietary staples. In the pantry, this means whole grains. The middle shelf contains things you eat only occasionally, like nonfat Greek yogurt, eggs, and low-fat cheese. The bottom shelf is restricted to just a couple of small treats. Once these are gone, that is all for the week. It may also help if you label your shelving by creating stickers. Whatever allows you to create a sound system is worth making it obvious.

Self-control is critical, and this system makes it easier than ever to not be tempted by opening the fridge and immediately seeing the rare treats rather than the staple foods. Your goal then should be to eat everything on your top shelf.

Chapter 5

How to Switch on Your Fitness and Exercise Habits

You do not need to become a dedicated super athlete to have a healthy exercise routine. Your goal should be to do a little bit of exercise every day to ensure you remain active and develop positive fitness habits. Not exercising can cause health impacts from weight gain to weakening muscles, bones (osteoporosis) and loss of elasticity of tendons & ligaments but as long as you stay active, you can reduce the risk of muscle atrophy (degeneration of muscle) and keep your strength up as you age. On top of direct physical benefits, exercise can have significant mental benefits as well. It can help you feel more energetic, refreshed and less stressed. With all these benefits, finding a little time to work out throughout the day is a no-brainer. Consistency is more important than how strenuous the workout is, so pick exercises that don't put too much strain on you and fit well into your typical schedule and lifestyle.

They Have It All Wrong! - Why Pain Doesn't Equal Gain

Fitness shouldn't be painful unless you are specifically training for an event and need to 'stretch' beyond your usual comfort zone. This doesn't mean you should never work up a sweat and be 'uncomfortable' at times, but it does mean that you don't have to risk exhaustion or injury to get healthy. Trying to push yourself too hard too fast can lead to an unsustainable workout schedule. Instead, stick to the mini habit's method. I recommend knowing your starting point, and this way you can pick the activities that are comfortable, realistic and suitable for you, and build slowly at a pace that feels right. If you don't think you could jog for 20 minutes, start with just five minutes and build your way up to longer jogs. It is admirable to decide you want to improve your fitness for any reason be it for an event, a health scare or increasing weight. I therefore want you to start slowly, build a solid base and progress with a sensible and long-term approach. I see too many people that try to hit the ground running, rather than starting at a slow walk and getting faster over time. This approach often can lead to giving up when lofty goals are not met. If you increase incrementally and start where you are comfortable, you are much more likely to continue the habit and enjoy the journey to your health and fitness goals.

January is a huge month for gyms, so much so that

"in a 2017 survey of nearly 6,400 fitness clubs in the U.S., the International Health, Racquet & Sports club Association found that 10.8 percent of all gym membership sales in 2016 took place in January, which is proportionally more than any other month that year" (Poon, 2019, para. 6). This makes January gym memberships seem like a great idea at first, as there is a big cultural push, but fitness is not seasonal, and many of the people who boast about their new resolutions don't even make it to February. The unfortunate truth is that fewer than 10% of the January rush will maintain their gym visits after the first three months. This is in part because these sorts of resolutions are rarely well-planned. They are hardly thought about during the feasting of the winter holidays, and once the initial enthusiasm wears off, people lose interest without a solid plan. Again, if you do not know your ideal outcome and the steps to reach it, how can you tell if your efforts are making a difference? By mid-January, many people exhaust themselves, lose their motivation when they don't see immediate results, and simply give up.

Why People Give Up On Exercise

Many health institutions rightly point out that people need to change their health habits, but simply saying this and not giving people the tools and mindset they need to succeed can be a narrow-minded approach. To understand how to stick with exercise past January, we must first understand why so many people aren't willing to keep working out.

1. They don't develop a plan

It is critical to know what your goals are and the frequency you expect yourself to exercise, or you cannot hold yourself accountable for these goals. More importantly, your reason for exercise needs to be compelling enough that it enables you to power through the desire to quit.

2. They are in a rush for immediate results

Many people I have consulted with believe they need to hit their top speed on day one. This idea is reinforced by exposure to shows like The Biggest Loser, which has contestants dragging tractor tires on the first day and collapsing due to exhaustion, but this kind of exercise is unsustainable, and they have medical personnel on-site for a reason. This

Habit Switch is about the idea of small, sustainable change with a long-term view. Under no circumstances do I want you to attempt to start a long-term activity at top speed!

3. They don't accommodate for their age and ability

As we get older, whether we want to admit it or not, our body's limitations change. As an example, I used to be able to dunk a basketball in my 20's. I went to the courts with my son recently and tried to show off, and after some warm-ups, stretching, and a few attempts, I was lucky if I could get within four inches of the hoop with my fingertips, let alone my whole wrist. Needless to say, my son wasn't too impressed with his dad!

I would love to be capable of all the things I could do in my 20's, but it is better for my fitness to accept what I can still do rather than keep trying to do things I can't anymore. As we start moving towards 30 years of age and older, our range of motion (R.O.M) decreases around our joints, and our muscles and tendons don't have the elasticity or strength they used to. These limitations are even more evident if you try to push yourself too hard. By starting slow, you give yourself so much more opportunity to strengthen muscles that have been in 'hibernation' for a few years.

As an example, here's a typical scenario for someone who fails to accommodate for their ability and jumps into exercise too quickly:

1. They notice they are gaining weight and think, "I have to do something about this, and fast!"

2. They Google local gyms or fitness camps.

3. They pay their membership fees with every intention of going for the 12 months they signed up for.

4. They get to the first session. Their energy and enthusiasm is pumping.

5. They push themselves hard on the first session for an hour. It's painful, but they see others well in advance of their current fitness and try to emulate their pace.

6. They get home, feeling exhausted but great about the session.

7. They wake up the following morning, feeling very stiff and sore. They say, "No problem, it's just a bit of muscle soreness."

8. They go to their next session. This time, motivation has dropped, the weights feel a lot

heavier, and their muscles still feel sore. They push through the session, but it's only 50 minutes this time rather than the scheduled hour.

9. During the next day, they feel even worse, sore all over from the workout. Even lifting their arm to brush their teeth becomes a chore.

10. When the next session is scheduled, something comes up at work. They think, "That's okay; I'll do it next time."

11. The session after that, they begrudgingly grab their gear, but nothing seems exciting about this anymore. They look around and see people effortlessly lifting weights, and their confidence takes a big hit.

12. They arrive home, sit on the couch, and think, "Maybe I'll take a break until my muscles are less sore."

13. Despite their best intentions, they never seem to be able to return, even after the soreness has faded.

Pushing yourself too hard is a one-way ticket to scaring yourself off the practice of exercise. It is immeasurably better to attend 20 sessions of low-activity exercise in a month than two sessions of high-activity exercise.

1. *The activity isn't sustainable*

I'm a huge advocate for activities you can keep doing into your 60's and 70's like power walking, cycling, swimming, dancing, golf, water aerobics, or other low-impact exercises. If you're in your teens, 20's, and 30's, then, by all means, participate in higher impact activities, but making sure that at least some of your exercise is sustainable for years to come is a great way to focus on the long term without increasing your risk of injury.

2. *The activity isn't enjoyable*

You should be doing activities you find fun. Lighten up a jog with music, or replace it with a dance routine. Do yoga with a group of friends. Your ability to keep exercising is dependent on you enjoying what you do.

3. *The activity is too expensive*

Some activities involve start-up costs related to equipment or ongoing costs in the form of classes or gym memberships. If you cannot afford to keep paying for the activity, you are unlikely to stick with it. Luckily, there are many cheap or free alternatives you can do if the cost is a barrier of entry for you.

4. *They don't STOP>REVIEW>PIVOT and POWER*

Developing your plan is your number one step for success, but it is just as important to take time to review your progress. Periodically decide if anything needs to change and if you need to make adjustments, determine how they can be structured into your daily routine and then power forward.

How did I manage to achieve my goal of 1,000 sit-ups per week in less than 90 days?

1,000 sit-ups in a week sounds like a lot, but in practice, it is easier to implement than you may think. In fact, it is something I now enjoy and have integrated into my morning routine as I mentioned at the beginning of the book. I want to walk you through my own process of integrating this exercise into my daily habits so that you can see firsthand the benefits of incremental, consistent increases in the frequency that you exercise.

- *Implementation Phase Example*: Goal of 1,000 sit-ups each week
- *Identification*: I need to increase my core abdominal strength.
- *My Why*: I want to reduce the chances of lower back pain that plagued me in my mid to late '30s so I can continue to play with my children.
- *Three Day Implementation Plan*: Following my early morning walk and breakfast, I will do 10 sit-ups each day for the next three days. The long-term plan is to build up to 170 sit-ups per day, six days per week to exceed my target of 1,000 sit-ups.

Next, I needed to make the process easy for myself. I needed to establish a cue for doing this activity that would encourage me to get it done every day.

1. I had an old yoga mat I hadn't used for ages, under my bed collecting dust. I brought it into the kitchen and rolled it up and placed it next to the dishwasher. I made sure it was easily accessible so I had somewhere comfortable to do my sit-ups.

2. To ensure I had my cue, I laid the yoga mat out on the floor before I left for my walk, as I'd have to literally walk over it when I came back.

3. I arrived back from my walk, had breakfast, and then as I walked back into the kitchen with my breakfast bowl, the yoga mat was right there.

4. I then completed 10 sit-ups and repeated this pattern for three days in a row. It wasn't enough to make me feel sore, but I had effectively laid the groundwork for a solid structure and a helpful reminder of my goal.

5. At my three-day review, I then planned that each day I would increase my sit-ups incrementally by three extra each day. When I reached 20, I would then split my sit-ups into sets of 10 with a rest in between.

6. Over the next 30 days, I then slowly increased my sit-ups by two each day. On Monday mornings, I increased by five, then reverted to increments of two for the rest of the week. As I progressed, I made sure I was doing sets of 15 or 20 at a time rather than doing them all at once.

My weekly goal plan to achieve 170 Sit-ups p/day

	MON	TUES	WED	THU	FRI	SAT	Rest Day
Week 1	10	12	14	16	18	20	
Week 2	25	27	29	31	33	35	
Week 3	40	42	44	46	48	50	
Week 4	55	57	59	61	63	65	

	MON	TUES	WED	THU	FRI	SAT	Rest Day
Week 5	70	72	74	76	78	80	
Week 6	85	87	89	91	93	95	
Week 7	100	102	104	106	108	110	
Week 8	115	117	119	121	123	125	

	MON	TUES	WED	THU	FRI	SAT	Rest Day
Week 9	130	132	134	136	138	140	
Week 10	145	147	149	151	153	155	
Week 11	160	162	164	166	168	170	

As this process demonstrates, I simply started small by developing my system and making progress easy. I now do over 4,000 sit-ups a month. This equates to 48,000 per year! If I had started by trying to do 70-100 sit-ups a day, I would have been sore and risked an abdominal strain, which might have made me give up altogether. Now I am capable of doing that many without much strain because I have slowly built up to it. You will also notice I included a rest day in my schedule, which is imperative as a reward system and as also recovery and repair for my abdominals. If I want to continue to increase my sit-ups, I would give myself two rest days to compensate. You can apply the above structure to any exercise or fitness habit you want to implement into your own life.

Don't Aim for Elite Fitness

Unless you are aiming to be the next big thing in the fitness world, you don't have to train like an elite athlete. I would recommend that you don't, and you instead stick to fitness habits that suit your lifestyle and capabilities. The definition by Segen's Medical Dictionary of an elite athlete is one who is considered to be "a person who is currently or has previously competed as a varsity player (individual or team), a professional player or a national or international level player". Chances are you are just trying to get your health up, so if you are not a professional athlete, why try to mirror the exercise habits of Olympians?

Keep in mind that elite athletes are under the supervision of personal trainers and coaches that know how hard they can push. They also have access to medical aid should it be required. Trying to become elite can be dangerous with or without the right resources. This book isn't trying to help you rise to the top of your exercise field; I only want to help you establish habits that you can integrate into a 40-60 hour work week, not ones that take a full-time commitment.

Your aim should be to develop a level of fitness that

best suits your goals and preferred outcomes. This means worrying about the long term too. There are very few sports that athletes are in for more than 15 years, with some even less than that. This is not sustainable, nor is it achievable on a regular schedule. Try to stick to habits that you can continue to complete for decades and whether you are working, on vacation, or even travelling for work.

The Seven Tips to Implement Your Habit Plan: How to Master a Fitness Plan for the Long Term

There are seven main tips to keep in mind so you can ensure you have all the knowledge you need to establish a fitness plan that lasts. These serve to summarize the chapter and give you simple, concise steps you can follow. If you master these tips, you will be in control of your physical health.

Healthy Fitness Step 1

Write down your five-year fitness goal

Writing down your five-year goal gives you a long-term focus rather than a short-term one. Once your five-year goal has been established, break that down into smaller steps and goals to achieve. I recommend you start each habit with the three-day trial run.

Setting fitness goals is a fantastic way to remain motivated. Your short-term fitness goals provide you with a close, relatively easy target to focus on, and you build your self-confidence while in the process. Your long-term goals keep your overall objective in the front of your mind, pushing you to keep exercising every day. When you reach your goals, check them off on your list and make new ones so you can continue moving forward.

Healthy Fitness Step 2

Fitness should be fun, not a chore

If you love your workout, it will never feel like a chore. Pick exercises that make you legitimately excited to get active. This will help keep you from dropping your routine. You should look forward to hitting the gym, going for a power walk or taking a jog, not dread it. When you're having fun, you won't have time to worry about these fears that could otherwise hold you back.

Healthy Fitness Step 3

Be very mindful of the ongoing expense of your fitness activity

If costs get too high, they can discourage you from continuing with your plan. Equipment, memberships, transportation, and travel costs can add up and make your exercise plan unsustainable. To avoid this, determine what the upfront costs for your exercise plan are and then look at the 12-month costs to see if you could keep up with them. Try to do 30-60 day trials first to ensure you really want to pay for a product or service. I'm sure there are many people with expensive road bikes, golf clubs, exercise bikes, 12-month gym memberships, and kayaks sitting unused in a garage or closet, gathering dust. Avoid making any ultimately unnecessary purchases.

Healthy Fitness Step 4

Build your fitness slowly - your body will thank you for it!

As mentioned previously, small steps are key. Build momentum with consistent change, frequent repetition, and structure while always keeping long-term benefits in mind. If you choose to go 0-

100 right out of the gate, you risk early burnout, lethargy, despondency, injury, and other potential health consequences.

Healthy Fitness Step 5

Fuel your body with the right foods to maintain energy

You may have every intention of developing a solid fitness plan and exercise habits, but if you don't have the diet to back it up, it will fall through. You need to ensure you are getting enough fuel and the right kind of energy for your workouts. Many people are willing to feed their car with premium gasoline to get better performance, but they do not realize that the same rule applies to their own body in the form of their diet. Give yourself the premium fuel you need to succeed.

Healthy Fitness Step 6

Have a Fitness Accountability Partner

Your Fitness Accountability Partner is someone who helps ensure you are staying on track. This person or group can be a friend, spouse, colleague, coach, or anyone that will encourage you to reach your goals. This system works particularly well when you have a training partner to keep you accountable for your exercise. In this circumstance, they may also need your support and aid when they are struggling through rough stages themselves. Lean on each other and share the experience of lifelong fitness as you exercise together.

Healthy Fitness Step 7

Be organized and create the least resistance

When implementing habits for exercise and diet, some habits may be more difficult than others. Make them as easy as possible to adopt by creating the lowest resistance to starting. Keep your habits small until you know you can do them. You may want to arrange things the night prior to starting a habit, so you have fewer reasons not to do it the next day. It also means having a specific time set for exercise. Structure will aid you immensely.

My personal example for my morning walks:

1. Before going to bed each night, I get my exercise gear ready. This way, I'm not fumbling around in the dark to get what I need.

2. I pre-set my podcast so I can just hit play.

3. The dog leash is ready at the back door.

By getting all of this done the night before, getting ready to exercise only involves getting out of bed and getting dressed.

For additional motivation, check out the Canadian Medical Association Journal study "[Health Benefits of Physical Activity: The Evidence](#)." It contains a breakdown of the benefits of exercise, which include a direct relationship with reducing cardiovascular disease and a wide variety of other conditions, including diabetes mellitus; cancer, namely colon and breast cancer; obesity; hypertension; bone and joint diseases like osteoporosis and osteoarthritis; and depression.

Chapter 6

Avoiding a Habit

Short-Circuit

A habit short circuit occurs when you are unable to keep pace with the habits you have established for yourself. You begin to slip behind, taking days off that turn into weeks and then months, all while promising you will get back to work soon but having no real intention of doing so. When troubles arise, such as old bad habits rearing their heads, you need to know how to efficiently tackle them and get back into the swing of things. You also need to know how to keep this habit short circuit from happening in the first place. This involves sticking to incremental change rather than large leaps, accepting your own limitations, working with others to achieve your goal, and most importantly knowing your motivation. I will break down these methods for dodging habit short circuits below.

When Bad Habits Re-Emerge

You are very likely to slip back into a bad habit or two at some point. What may start as a single instance of breaking your diet or fitness routine can quickly spiral out of hand. If you don't have a strong enough reason behind your desire for change, you may not be able to resist these bad habits when they appear. If you feel strongly about kicking the poor habits, you can start to understand why this relapse occurs so you can prevent it next time. Ask yourself, "Was there any particular event or feeling you had that triggered this change of mindset? Was there a particular event in your life that caused a change in structure?" Understanding the real cause of returning to negative habits can shed light on the common triggers preceding each instance of relapse. Identifying these triggers helps you become more aware of your weak points. So, how can you get back on track?

Revisit Your Schedule

Your weak point may be in your schedule. If you cannot reliably stick to your schedule, either because it is too packed or too loose, you will start to make excuses for not following it. My morning habits are heavily disciplined, which means I know I can get all of my morning habits done on time. Adopting a schedule with a similar level of structure can help ensure you don't procrastinate on your goals. Rework your schedule until it fits your life.

Use Existing Momentum

Use the success and momentum you have built up with other habits to get those that have slipped back on track. Don't waste time doing the habit equivalent of staring at a blank page, waiting for words to come. Start working on adjacent goals and use the progress you make on those to revisit the habits that stumped you. Succeeding at integrating a habit boosts your self-confidence, which gives you the burst of positivity you need to tackle tougher habits.

Don't Miss More Than Two Days

Taking long breaks between your habits can cause them to fade out of your body's memory. Staying consistent is especially important during the early phases of building a habit, as taking breaks longer than 48 hours can start to weaken the links that turn habits into an automatic process. If you need to rest, it is better to take two non-consecutive days off.

Make Your Environment Conducive to Success

Environmental factors can play an important role in

either keeping your motivated or aiding distraction and the return of bad habits. If you still have a cabinet full of high fat and high sugar foods, you will be tempted to break your healthy eating habits every time you open the pantry. If you keep the TV on while you work, you may spend more time watching it than getting anything done. I like getting up early to read and exercise as it is such a quiet and peaceful time with relatively few distractions. Figure out what your ideal environment is and take steps to make your surroundings match.

Your environment does not just mean physical space. It also refers to the music and media you listen to that can impact your energy levels, as well as the people you surround yourself with. If those close to you are frequently encouraging you to make bad choices, preventing you from keeping your habits or even forcing you to change something you do not feel similarly passionate about changing, you may need to reevaluate who you spend time with. Fill your life with people and things that support your goals, and you will find it much easier to keep your good habits around.

Mix Things Up

Try things out and see what works, and if one thing doesn't work, swap it for something else. Make improving your fitness an adventure and use it as an excuse to try new things. Above all else, don't constrain yourself to my schedule or anyone else's. What works for me or anyone else may not necessarily fit your schedule, lifestyle, or environment. Never try to conform to the schedule and habits of someone else if it does not positively impact you to do so. Try different schedules and routines until, and you find the one that works for you.

Revisit Your Goals to Ensure Alignment

The more time you spend writing down, reading, and reviewing your goals, the more they are programmed into your subconscious. Make sure your goals still align with what you want in life one month, six months, five years, and even ten years after setting them. Some recommend doing this review process every morning during what is called the "Golden Hour," or the first hour you are awake. This is the perfect time to revisit your goals because "the things that you do in the first hour prepare your mind and set you up for the entire day. During the first thirty to sixty minutes, take time to think and review your plans for the future" (Tracy, n.d.-b, para. 3). Getting a good start and reiterating the importance of your goals makes those goals stand out more as you go about the rest of the day.

The Resilience Factor

Resiliency can help you bounce back after even the toughest of stumbling blocks. Each time you forge ahead after a setback, you improve your resilience. The decision to keep going will help you continue to build positive habits even when they become hard to maintain. Change can be difficult, so don't expect everything to be smooth sailing. The question is not whether you will struggle or pass with flying colors; the question is whether or not you will pick yourself up, dust yourself off, and keep moving after a setback occurs.

Reward and Celebration – The Goal Loop

One area I have yet to discuss is the celebration after a victory. When you have achieved success, small or large, take time to celebrate it. Little rewards can boost your morale and encourage you to keep moving.

To enable my clients to have a visual of what this celebration looks like, I designed the 'GOAL LOOP' system as outlined in my book Magnetic Goals.

Below is an excerpt from this book to highlight the importance of celebration.

The Purpose of the Goal Loop

The goal loop provides a concrete, cyclical structure for all of your goal progress. It operates on the principles of rhythm, repetition, structure, clarity, and action. The phases allow you to develop a familiar rhythm of goal setting and achieving with positive feedback in the form of celebrating at the end. Because the phases loop back on themselves, they use repetition to encourage you to complete future goals. This process is similar to the repetition involved in daily habits which cause them to feel second nature after you have had enough practice incorporating them into your life. The goal loop is structured with an easy to follow path, so you always know what the next step is, and there is no opportunity to waste precious time. It provides you with clarity on your next move and how to achieve what you have always wanted. Most important of all, it encourages perpetual action rather than stagnation. Once one goal is accomplished, it is time to move onto the next. If you keep moving, there is nothing you cannot achieve. The beauty of The Goal Loop is that each time you complete the cycle, your goal setting structure and systems gain strength and become extremely robust.

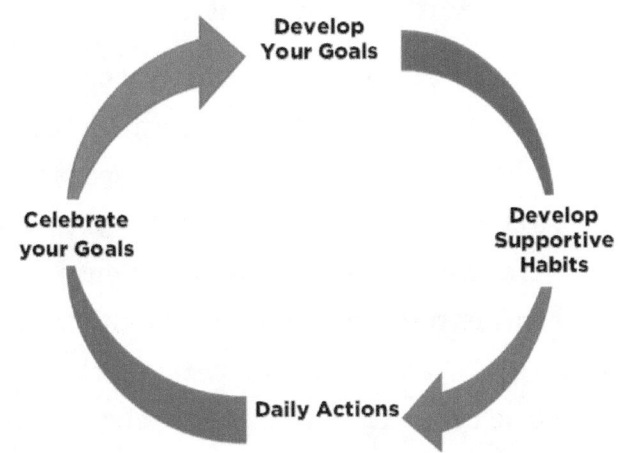

Cyclical Phases

The goal loop is broken up into four phases, each of which reflects a previously discussed aspect of the goal setting and achieving process.

Phase One is establishing your goals. Use this time to understand what you want to accomplish. *Phase*

Two is the development of supportive daily habits that will help you get where you want to go. In *Phase Three*, you will take daily actions that propel you towards success. These phases culminate in achieving your goals, celebrating, and starting the goal loop anew armed with the knowledge you have learned from your last cycle.

Phase One: Setting Your Goals

Goal setting is the foundation of every cycle of goal achievement. Each time you return to the goal-setting phase, consider what you have learned from the last cycle. What goals worked for you? Which ones were easy to stick to, and which ones did you have a harder time finding the right motivation for? Are the goals you are setting in this cycle, helping you to reach your 12-month goals, or have your 12-month goals changed? You should also be re-examining your *why factor* in this phase and making sure you still feel dedicated to the goals you set. Coming up with a powerful, solid set of goals that you feel passionately about in Phase One lays the foundation for the next phases and paves the way for future successes.

Phase Two: Establishing Supportive Daily Habits

You already know the amazing benefits that the right habits can have on your ability to achieve your goals. Knowing what works for you and what doesn't can help you revise and review your list of habits and identify which habits you can continue including in your schedule and which need to change. Update any habits that are specific to goals that have already been achieved to reflect your new ones. For example, if you have accomplished your first goal of weight loss and your new goal is developing muscle tone, you may need to establish a new workout routine to achieve different results. When reviewing your already existing daily habits and creating new ones, ask yourself the following questions. How is this habit helping me to achieve my current goals? Is there any new information I should direct my focus on learning? What habits were hardest to stick to last time, and why? How can I either modify these habits to make them more suited to my lifestyle and enjoyable? Answering these questions can help you keep your daily habits aligned as closely as possible to your goals.

Phase Three: Daily Action

Phase Three is about acting on the goals you have set and the habits you have chosen and taking actions every day that move you closer to the finish line. Many of the actions you take for various goals may be the same with only slight differences. For example, whether you are looking to start a new business or write a book, you will need to do research; however, the type of research you will have to do to launch your business successfully is different from the information you will have to gather for your book. You can use the actions you have completed for past goals to form a blueprint for your current ones and make the appropriate modifications when necessary. Remember to start with small actions and build up to larger ones, but keep moving forward no matter what. Daily actions help you build momentum that will carry you through to current and future goals.

Phase Four: Achieving Your Goals and Celebrating

You've done it! You have remained committed and focused, and in exchange, you have done what you have set out to do. Completing your goals can help you to feel more fulfilled on top of the benefits they already provide. The gratification from knowing your time and energy has paid off is immense. Take some time to appreciate all the hard work you have put into your success. Do something to celebrate, as you should be proud of yourself. Just ensure that it is nothing that will tip you back into performing any negative habits that you have worked so hard to eradicate.

Next, it is time to roll all of these positive feelings into motivation to tackle your next goal. You are likely riding high on positive emotions, and by now, you have realized the extent of what you are capable of. Success is a very powerful motivator. Armed with the knowledge and the proof that when you truly apply yourself, you really can accomplish what once felt like a faraway dream, starting on your next dream is the natural next step. Turn this success into achieving another goal, and another, until you are working your way up to your big 3-year and 5-year goals. You already have the tools and experience to ensure you are successful; you just need to put them to use by returning to the goal-setting loop.

Decision Making with the Future in Mind

Following the path of The Goal Loop encourages you to think about your upcoming goals and your ideal future. It is a tool you can use to develop a plan that works for you and is unique to what you want to achieve while still being versatile enough to accommodate all of your goals. This means the decisions you make must also be forward-thinking as you consider what impact your choices have on your future.

Start establishing the goals you want to achieve as early as possible, so you have every possible opportunity to develop positive habits and guide your decisions in the areas you choose to focus on. If you understand the relationship between your choices, the goal loop, and the end result of your life, you can use critical turning point moments and crucial decisions to effectively alter your future.

Eradicate the Perfection Mindset

Trying to achieve perfection can be a detriment to your success. Perfect, by definition, means "complete and correct in every way, of the best possible type or without fault" (Cambridge Dictionary, n.d., para. 1). Placing the lofty expectations of being "without fault" on yourself only ensures that when you do inevitably have difficulties, as you are only human, you will be much harder on yourself than you would if you kept realistic expectations. If you "allow yourself to do things incompletely, imperfectly, and imprecisely," you will "progress to the state of completion and precision" (Chua, n.d., para. 13) rather than getting bogged down in ensuring everything is perfect. It is better to get two 90% grades than one 100% and one 0% because you weren't able to move on from the first assignment. You may even be able to use your experience completing both tasks to get better at future ones.

Of course, if social media posts are to be believed, perfect people are everywhere. However, these posts are entirely curated to suggest this; you don't see the hundreds of failed attempts, only a single success. Additionally, not everyone's idea of perfection will align, making it even more of an impossible goal. Don't let yourself be deceived by these unachievable ideals.

Escaping perfectionism

Perfectionism can create additional hurdles that keep you standing still. You may never feel like you are finished with a task, or you may constantly feel stressed about your performance. You aren't able to build your skills incrementally because you are so fixated on getting to 100% as fast as possible. It can also impact your ability to try new things. If you constantly fear failure "you often adopt a mindset of, *If I can't do it perfectly, then I won't even try* [...] In essence, your fear of failure actually makes you fail" (Lombardo, 2017, para. 6). Improving your overall health is often dependent on your ability to try something new and take a risk that just might pay off.

If you are a perfectionist, how do you let go of the need to always be perfect? For one, get comfortable with the idea of failure. If you accept failure as a natural part of an attempt rather than a forbidden outcome, you will be more inclined to put yourself out there. For another, start valuing your own goals, decisions, and successes whenever they occur. Many perfectionists are overly reliant on what others think of them. Once you learn to start caring more about your own opinion of yourself and valuing your input, your need to be perfect will begin to fade. Remember that when it comes to decision making in your own life, you are the authority on yourself, and therefore you do not need to be reliant on others to decide what is right for you (Cohen, 2018, para. 15). Self-confidence will help you minimize fears of failure and bolster your self-reliance.

Group Energy - The Power of Others

If you have difficulty staying committed when you're flying solo, try joining a group of likeminded people or making one yourself. This might mean joining a sports team, working out with friends, making a swimming squad, or joining an online group that allows you to share similar experiences and questions. Knowing that others are experiencing the same things you are and sharing tips and tricks will encourage you to keep going.

Group workouts are growing increasingly popular. A 2017 study suggests that when we exercise alongside our peers, we are more likely to attend class, put in the necessary effort, and even improve our mental state. Participants who attended at least one class a week saw "a statistically significant decrease in stress, and an improvement in the mental, physical, and emotional quality of life" (Knight, 2017, para. 15). If you want to enjoy every benefit fitness has to offer, group exercise is the way to go.

Group energy isn't just restricted to exercise. It can also help with dieting, as "one study found that 95 percent of those who started a weight-loss program with friends completed the program, compared to a 76 percent completion rate for those who tackled the program alone" (Steinhilber, 2017, para. 9). If you have others to lean on, you will find yourself more committed to hitting your goals and sticking to your habits. This is the power of support from a group.

Link It Back to Your Two Why's

All outcomes we achieve ultimately come back to two things. The first is the decisions we make, and the second is the actions we take. When you make a choice or take action, you may ask yourself, "Why did I make that decision? What is the underlying reason?" A strong desire can positively influence your decisions, while uncertainty in your goals will make good decisions harder to make.

If you find that you are regularly slipping back into bad habits, you need to determine your two 'why's. The first 'why' is why you make the choices you do, as well as how they are either positively or negatively impacting you. What is the driving motivation behind your decisions, and if it is a negative factor, what should you do to make it a positive force? The second 'why' is why you need to implement a given change. How will the change impact your long-term health?

If you are having trouble understanding your motivations, I highly recommend the "Why?" section of Luke Bremner's article "The Importance Of Understanding The 'Why' Behind Your Goals." Being in tune with and in control of your motivations will let you move forward and avoid the habit short circuit.

Chapter 7

Implement
and
Take Action

You have all the knowledge you will need to achieve success. You understand the theory behind mini habits and the amazing effect they can have on your life, as well as how to put them into practice. The only thing left for you to do is take the necessary steps to implement what you have read into your own life. Reading and collecting knowledge is great, but if you never put that knowledge into practice, you will never be able to see any change. You might read every book on basketball in the world, but if you never attempt to a 3 pointer you can hardly call yourself a basketball master.

Many people make the mistake of simply learning and not doing. They assure themselves they will start, soon, but as the weeks and months go on, they lose the initial burst of motivation they had when they finished listening to a podcast episode or reading a book. By the time they get around to starting, they have forgotten everything they have read. The only way around this is by taking action and getting in practice as soon as possible. Starting to apply what you have read will reinforce what you've learned. You need to shift from being a huge consumer of books, audio and seminars and begin to pause and take action on those things that resonated with you, otherwise, you're much more likely to forget 90% of the material. There is no better time to start putting what you read and listen to into practice than right now.

If you find some aspect of the habit switch process slips your memory, review it as often as you need. Take notes and highlight what speaks to you. Discussing the ideas in the book with friends can help keep them fresh, and you may even convert them into a partner on your quest for better health. Involving friends can also help you get a better angle on what you have read. If you have a friend who tends to tackle problems in a different way, discussing your new plan as outlined in *The Habit Switch* with them can provide you with a new point of view and additional insights on what you have read. You may end up seeing an idea in a whole new light.

You are ready to begin the journey to a healthier, happier life. All it takes is employing the strategies you have already learned. If you can take action, you should; that is, if you feel you can make a change or implement something, then do it now. Hold yourself accountable for getting started as soon as you can. You cannot put your health on the backburner.

Actionable Items

If you are committed to getting moving right away, here are some specific, actionable items you can do right now to get started. They will make the transition from learning to doing easier and supply you with a roadmap for success.

Highlight what matters

What sections stood out to you most? Which really gave you that extra push of motivation, or provided a suggestion you would like to implement? Return to these sections and highlight the lines that really matter to you. When you return to the book in the future, you can easily find the ideas that sparked your passion and drive without necessarily needing to reread every sentence. In may only take you 10 minutes, but these reflection points will be highly valuable for you in the years to come.

Write out your goals

Figure out what goals matter most to you and start writing them down. Start with the big-ticket items, and then consider the smaller day-to-day goals you want to achieve. What habits would you need to adopt to reach your goals? What implementation strategy works best for achieving these outcomes?

Once you have written out your goals, you should have a real plan you can follow.

Introduce your first goal

Start small! It is the key message of this book and the one thing I hope you keep in mind when putting my strategies into practice. Small changes lead to a big impact. Choose just one goal and give it the three-day test run. Decide what you like and what isn't working for you, rework, and try again. Don't try to introduce additional goals and habits for achieving them until you feel like you have fully integrated the first habit into your schedule. This will prevent you from overburdening yourself and give the new habit time to work its magic so you can take notice of its results.

Keep building

Increase the frequency and, slowly, the number of your habits until you are creeping closer to your goals. Continue to build off past successes and keep moving. If you stick with it and keep up your habits for health, you really can achieve a healthier body and mind.

Conclusion

Your fitness determines so many other aspects of your future. If you don't keep your body in good shape, you will not be able to experience so much of what life has to offer. Health issues resulting from poor fitness habits limit your ability to live up to your full potential. You may miss out on opportunities, be unable to perform certain tasks, or experience increased stress and other mental health woes. Your body is the vehicle by which you make your way through life, and you deserve a body that is as reliable as you need it to be.

When you prioritize your health, you unlock so many pathways that might have otherwise been barred to you. Healthy eating gives you energy, helps you manage your weight, and ensures that your body will function at full capacity. Healthy exercise builds up your strength, helps discourage weight gain, and keeps you fit long into your life. You can ensure huge future success just by taking small steps today. If you set up the right habits now, they will stay with you for 20, 30, and even 50 years down the line. Set the precedent for good health habits early and save yourself trouble in the long run.

The Power of Small

Every choice you make has an impact. Simple incremental changes and positive decisions build-up to a landslide effect. Actions that seem small in isolation, like taking a power walk through the park or drinking the daily recommended dose of water, are not so small when added up over years and years of good habits. A handful of pushups in the morning turns into hundreds, which turns into thousands, which turns into tens of thousands. If you convert an action into a habit by repeating it frequently and giving it time to grow, you will reap immense rewards.

Remember to always keep your long-term goals in mind. You won't see a change right away, but if you stick with the mini habits, you will need no help seeing the difference five years later. The difference that properly implemented mini habits can have on your life is enormous. If you need some help seeing this change early on, the STOP>REVIEW>PIVOT and POWER system is your friend.

Using Review to Your Advantage

Self-awareness is an extremely important skill for improving your health. With it, you can accurately determine which aspects of your plan are helping you and which ones aren't doing as much good as you had hoped. An honest review and acceptance of where you are, without guilt, can save you months of plugging away at an ineffective strategy.

This is where the *STOP>REVIEW>PIVOT* and *POWER* system comes into play. Use it to get a general grasp on how far you've come and where you need to go next. First, stop and take note of what you are currently doing. Then see if it is helping you achieve your specific goals. If not, pivot and adjust your habits. Finally, power on through with renewed confidence that what you are doing will get you closer to the outcome you want. With this system, you ensure that every step you take is one in the right direction. This allows you to make a positive change every single day.

Making Progress Every Day

True fitness is not about a sudden burst of activity or weight loss bookended by periods of lethargy. It is about establishing sustainable habits that set you up for long-term success. Habits ensure that you never go a day without making some kind of progress, big or small - and of course, even small progress is success unfolding at a sustainable rate. Picture your habits like a school of fish. One fish alone is not much to look at, but start multiplying that fish to hundreds, maybe even thousands more, and suddenly you have one very big school. Completing your daily habits is like adding another fish to the school, knowing that given enough time you will have something really notable on your hands.

Goal achievement and daily habits are intricately linked. You cannot have one without the other. Trying to establish habits without knowing what they are for or why you even want to bother pursuing them will leave you headed in multiple different directions at once, never really narrowing your focus or expanding upon your habits in a positive way. You need goals to serve as the coordinates for your destination. Trying to reach your goals without habits is an equally impossible task. You cannot lose weight by exercising in the gym but then rewarding yourself with a bowl of confectionery or ice-cream at home. Your habits have to support what you want to achieve. You also cannot achieve your goals overnight, and you cannot expect anything done quickly to be sustainable; you need to build up habits so that they stick with you for years. You need to be committed for the long term and never expect short term gains. To be honest, the reward for some changes can take from 6 – 12 months just to see very small results. If you can successfully do this, which I firmly believe you can, you will make continual progress towards your goals and achieve outstanding results.

Input equals output

You need to look after your body. It is absolutely imperative for all other paths to success. Even if you do not do a lot of physical work now, you will find that as you get older, there will come a time where you will notice just how long it has been since you properly stretched your muscles and joints, which can make starting an exercise and weight loss plan much harder execute. You would not allow a boat to sit at port for months or years, completely without maintenance, and then try to take it out on the sea in the middle of a storm and expect to have a successful voyage. Treat your body with the same consideration. The maintenance and prep work you give to your body in the form of diet and exercise will keep you in top condition so you can be prepared for even the roughest of storms.

Health does not have to be a painful process, nor does it have to be an amazing sudden change. If you commit yourself to your habits every day, you can flip the habit switch on and jumpstart your progress towards attaining a healthy body and living a more fulfilling, healthy, and happy life.

To conclude, I wanted to leave you with this from the legendary Les Brown, US motivational speaker and author. I think he sums your potential up perfectly with this quote.

"I know something about you, even not knowing you, that you have greatness within you. You have the ability to do things that you can't even begin to imagine. You have talents and skills in you that you haven't even begun to reach for yet. When you are working at your dreams, people say, the harder the battle, the sweeter the victory. It's good because when the battle is hard, and you struggle, it's what you become in the process that is more important. It's the kind of person you become, the character that you build, the courage that you develop, the faith that you manifest. It's great when you wake up in the morning, and you look yourself in the mirror, and you're a different kind of person. You walk with a different kind of spirit. It doesn't matter what happens to you; what matters is what you are going to do about it! Easy is not an option."

I know you can do this because you are now equipped with the knowledge, the steps and the systems to make a significant change in your life. It's time to turn on **The Habit Switch**!

PLEASE LEAVE A REVIEW

I would greatly appreciate if you enjoyed this book to leave a review on Amazon. Reviews will assist **The Habit Switch** to reach more people for a positive impact on their lives.

You may also be interested in joining the EXCLUSIVE Review Team to receive future books in return for leaving an honest review.

To leave a review, please visit www.amazon.com

To be part of the **Exclusive Book Review** Team, please visit www.thelifegraduate.com and go to the contact tab on the website.

ABOUT THE AUTHOR

Romney is the founder of The Life Graduate and author of 6 books including **Magnetic Goals**, **The Daily Goal Tracker** and **Job Launch**.

He has represented Australia in the World Championships in Dragon Boat Racing, he is a business coach, motivational speaker, qualified teacher, author and owner of two rapidly growing businesses in the educational space.

Romney has dedicated the past 20 years to helping others achieve success and fulfillment in their lives through his coaching, teaching, masterclasses, mentoring, resources and books. His clients speak of his passion and dedication for self-improvement and bringing that knowledge and experience to help others achieve what they want in their lives.

He is a sought-after speaker and is regarded as one of the leading experts in goal setting and daily habits with the development of the unique Dr. ACTION™ and 'The Goal Loop' systems. He has a Bachelor of Education in Physical Education, is a qualified Personal Trainer and has previously held Head of Faculty positions in some of the most prestigious schools in Australia. He has also held senior executive positions in leading growth companies and currently has an advisory role at Australia's largest provider of mobile dental to schools.

Romney and his wife have two children along with their pet dog, Ruby. He is a passionate and avid golfer and spends his vacations at some of the most picturesque seaside locations in Victoria and Queensland in Australia.

Please refer to the below details to reach out to Romney for speaking engagements, podcasts or other media requests.

Web. www.thelifegraduate.com

LinkedIn. Romney Nelson

Other books by the Author

Magnetic Goals

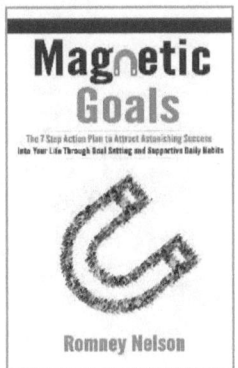

Available in Hardcopy, Audiobook and eBook.

The Daily Goal Tracker (Journal)
Testimonial by Brian Tracy

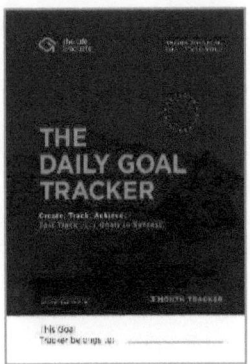

Hardcopy Only

Job Launch

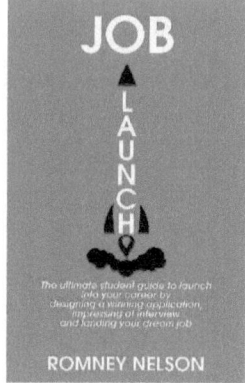

Available in Hardcopy, Audiobook and eBook

Resources

A.D.A.M. (2018, April 23). Facts about polyunsaturated fats. Retrieved February 16, 2020, from https://medlineplus.gov/ency/patientinstructions/000747.htm

Altrogge, S. (2019, April 30). 12 Morning and Evening Routines That Will Set Up Each Day for Success. Retrieved February 16, 2020, from https://zapier.com/blog/daily-routines/

American Academy of Family Physicians. (2017, March 27). Hydration: Why It's So Important. Retrieved February 16, 2020, from https://familydoctor.org/hydration-why-its-so-important/

American Academy of Family Physicians. (2019, July 22). Vegetarian Diet: How to Get the Nutrients You Need. Retrieved February 16, 2020, from https://familydoctor.org/vegetarian-diet-how-to-get-the-nutrients-you-need/

Barradell, S., Ennals, P., Burnett, M., Murphy, F., Karasmanis, S., & Connors, A. (2019, February 20). Reflective practice in health. Retrieved February 16, 2020, from https://latrobe.libguides.com/reflectivepractice

Beer, S. (2019, September 30). Why seasonal diets could be the answer to food sustainability. Retrieved February 16, 2020, from

https://www.independent.co.uk/news/health/seasonal-diets-food-sustainability-climate-change-crisis-a9116981.html

Better Health Channel. (2012, October). Vegetarian and vegan eating. Retrieved February 16, 2020, from https://www.betterhealth.vic.gov.au/health/healthyliving/vegetarian-and-vegan-eating

Better Health Channel. (2015, June). Physical activity – Setting yourself goals. Retrieved February 16, 2020, from https://www.betterhealth.vic.gov.au/health/healthyliving/physical-activity-setting-yourself-goals

Bjarnadottir, A. (2019, January 3). 9 Popular Weight Loss Diets Reviewed. Retrieved February 16, 2020, from https://www.healthline.com/nutrition/9-weight-loss-diets-reviewed

Breene, S. (2013, October 7). 13 Unexpected Benefits of Exercise. Retrieved February 16, 2020, from https://greatist.com/fitness/13-awesome-mental-health-benefits

Briggs, S. (2015, February 10). 25 Ways to Develop a Growth Mindset. Retrieved February 16, 2020, from https://www.opencolleges.edu.au/informed/features/develop-a-growth-mindset/

Cambridge Dictionary. (n.d.). Transformational. Retrieved February 16, 2020, from https://dictionary.cambridge.org/dictionary/english/transformatio nal

Candelaria, K. B. (2016, April 6). Health Buzzwords: How Food Marketing Is Misleading You. Retrieved February 16, 2020, from http://www.fitnesshq.com/food-marketing/

Clear, J. (n.d.-a). How to Master the Art of Continuous Improvement. Retrieved February 16, 2020, from https://jamesclear.com/continuous-improvement

Clear, J. (n.d.-b). The 3 R's of Habit Change: How To Start New Habits That Actually Stick. Retrieved February 16, 2020, from https://jamesclear.com/three-steps-habit-change

Clear, J. (n.d.-c). Why Small Habits Make a Big Difference. Retrieved February 16, 2020, from https://fs.blog/2018/12/habits-james-clear/

Dallasnews Administrator. (2013, April 15). The dangers of salt and sugar - And how to protect yourself. Retrieved February 16, 2020, from https://www.dallasnews.com/news/healthy-living/2013/04/15/the-dangers-of-salt-and-sugar-and-how-to-protect-yourself/

Davis, L. (n.d.). Always looking forwards? It might be time to reflect. Retrieved February 16, 2020, from https://this.deakin.edu.au/self-improvement/always-looking-forwards-it-might-be-time-to-reflect

EvolutionEat. (2017, February 24). Fixed Mindset vs Growth Mindset. Retrieved February 16, 2020, from https://evolutioneat.com/fixed-mindset-vs-growth-mindset/

Foroux, D. (n.d.). The Power Of Compounding: You Can Achieve Anything, If You Stop Trying To Do Everything. Retrieved February 16, 2020, from https://dariusforoux.com/the-power-of-compounding/

Frost-Sharratt, C. (n.d.). Eating Habits Learned in Childhood are Not All Good. Retrieved February 16, 2020, from https://www.weightlossresources.co.uk/food/behaviour-eating-habits.htm

Gardner, B., Lally, P., & Wardle, J. (2012). Making health habitual: The psychology of 'habit-formation' and general practice. *British Journal of General Practice*, 62(605), 664–666. doi: 10.3399/bjgp12X659466

Gardner, B., & Rebar, A. L. (2019, January 15). Habit Formation and Behavior Change. Retrieved from https://www.oxfordbibliographies.com/view/document/obo-9780199828340/obo-9780199828340-0232.xml

Good Magazine. (n.d.). We are what we eat. Retrieved February 16, 2020, from https://good.net.nz/article/we-are-what-we-eat

Gunnars, K. (2018, July 25). Intermittent Fasting 101 - The Ultimate Beginner's Guide. Retrieved February 16, 2020, from https://www.healthline.com/nutrition/intermittent-fasting-guide

Gunnars, K. (2018, May 23). Why Is Fiber Good for You? The Crunchy Truth. Retrieved February 16, 2020, from https://www.healthline.com/nutrition/why-is-fiber-good-for-you

Hall, S. H. (2016, October 25). Why writing down your 3 MIT's at night can change your life. Retrieved February 16, 2020, from https://www.onepagecrm.com/blog/make-time-change-life/

Harvard Healthbeat. (n.d.). 7 ways to jumpstart healthy change in your life. Retrieved February 16, 2020, from https://www.health.harvard.edu/healthbeat/7-ways-to-jumpstart-healthy-change-in-your-life

Heart UK. (n.d.). Saturated fat. Retrieved February 16, 2020, from https://www.heartuk.org.uk/low-cholesterol-foods/saturated-fat

Heijligers, H. (n.d.). Don't expect results too quickly (GrowthMindset

Hacks Series). Retrieved February 16, 2020, from https://smartleadershiphut.com/growth-mindset/expect-results-quickly/

Hills, A. P., Byrne, N. M., Lindstrom, R., & Hill, J. O. (2013). 'Small Changes' to Diet and Physical Activity Behaviors for Weight Management. *Obesity Facts*, 6(3), 228–238. doi:10.1159/000345030

Holland, K. (2019, January 8). Your Body Wants It — How Adopting a 'Seasonal Diet' Can Make You Healthier. Retrieved February 16, 2020, from https://www.healthline.com/health-news/adopting-a-seasonal-diet-may-help-you-lose-weight#How-seasonal-eating-works

Knight, C. (2017, November 21). Group workouts shown to improve mental & physical wellbeing. Retrieved February 16, 2020, from https://www.lesmills.com/uk/fit-planet/fitness/group-exercise-research/

Kullar, P. S. (2016, July 31). 1% a day makes you 37 times better in a year. Retrieved February 16, 2020, from https://medium.com/life-maths/life-maths-1-change-a-day-make-you-37-times-better-in-1-year-eeb66db70120

Marcin, A. (2018, December 7). Are You a Healthy Weight? Weight Ranges by Height and Sex. Retrieved February 16, 2020, from https://www.healthline.com/health/how-much-should-i-weigh#bmi

Mawer, R. (2018, July 30). The Ketogenic Diet: A Detailed Beginner's Guide to Keto. Retrieved February 16, 2020, from https://www.healthline.com/nutrition/ketogenic-diet-101

Mayo Clinic Staff. (2017, August 16). Atkins Diet: What's behind the claims? Retrieved February 16, 2020, from https://www.mayoclinic.org/healthy-lifestyle/weight-loss/in-depth/atkins-diet/art-20048485

McKenna. (2019, February 2). 8 Reasons To Commit To A Healthy Lifestyle. Retrieved February 16, 2020, from https://wedtowellness.com/8-reasons-to-commit-to-a-healthy-lifestyle/

Muttucumaru, A. (2018, March 1). Why eating what's in season is good for you - and how to eat well. Retrieved February 16, 2020, from https://www.getthegloss.com/article/what-s-in-season-how-to-eat-well-all-year-round

NutritionED. (n.d.). Types of Diets. Retrieved February 16, 2020, from https://www.nutritioned.org/types-of-diets.html

Poon, L. (2019, January 16). The Rise and Fall of New Year's Fitness Resolutions, in 5 Charts. Retrieved February 16, 2020, from https://www.citylab.com/life/2019/01/do-people-keep-new-years-resolution-fitness-weight-loss-data/579388/

Sample, I. (2018, April 30). The five habits that can add more than a decade to your life. Retrieved February 16, 2020, from https://www.theguardian.com/science/2018/apr/30/the-five-habits-that-can-add-more-than-a-decade-to-your-life

Sass, C. (2019, January 24). What Is the TLC Diet, and Can It Help You Lose Weight? A Nutritionist Explains. Retrieved February 16, 2020, from https://www.health.com/weight-loss/what-is-tlc-diet

Scuderi, R. (2019, October 15). How to Invest in Yourself: 3 Valuable Ways to Change Your Life. Retrieved February 16, 2020, from https://www.lifehack.org/articles/lifestyle/3-valuable-ways-to-invest-in-yourself.html

Segal, R., & Robinson, L. (2019, June). Choosing Healthy Fats. Retrieved February 16, 2020, from https://www.helpguide.org/articles/healthy-eating/choosing-healthy-fats.htm

Segen's Medical Dictionary. (2011). Elite Athlete. Retrieved February 16, 2020, from https://medical-dictionary.thefreedictionary.com/elite-athlete

Semeco, A. (2017, February 10). The Top 10 Benefits of Regular Exercise. Retrieved February 16, 2020, from https://www.healthline.com/nutrition/10-benefits-of-exercise

Settembre, J. (2018, January 21). This is the insane amount millennials are spending on fitness. Retrieved February 16, 2020, from https://www.marketwatch.com/story/this-is-the-insane-amount-millennials-are-spending-on-fitness-2018-01-21

Spies, D. (2018, April 6). 5 Tips To Create More Self Discipline for Health Weight Loss. Retrieved February 16, 2020, from https://cleananddelicious.com/5-tips-to-create-more-self-discipline-for-health-weight-loss/

Spritzler, F. (2016, December 20). 11 Impressive Health Benefits of Salmon. Retrieved February 16, 2020, from https://www.healthline.com/nutrition/11-benefits-of-salmon

Sreenivasan, S. (2017, December 15). 5 Signs That It's Time to Change Your Life's Direction. Retrieved February 16, 2020, from https://thriveglobal.com/stories/5-signs-that-it-s-time-to-change-your-life-s-direction/

Strengthminded_Erict. (2019, February 19). Misleading Claims in Health, Fitness, and Nutrition Advertising. Retrieved February 16, 2020, from https://www.strengthminded.com/misleading-claims-in-health-fitness-and-nutrition-advertising/

Tracy, B. (n.d.-a). 6 Reasons Setting Goals Is Important. Retrieved February 16, 2020, from https://www.briantracy.com/blog/personal-success/importance-of-goal-setting/

Tracy, B. (n.d.-b). The Golden Hour (Continued). Retrieved February 16, 2020, from https://www.briantracy.com/blog/general/the-golden-hour-2/

Tracy, B. (n.d.-c). Turn All Your Dreams Into Reality With A Personal Development Plan. Retrieved February 16, 2020, from https://www.briantracy.com/blog/personal-success/personal-development-plan/

Tull, M. (2017, December 6). Top 10 Ways to Invest in Yourself and Why It's So Powerful. Retrieved February 16, 2020, from https://www.huffpost.com/entry/top-10-ways-to-invest-in-_b_8406130

Guidelines for a Low Cholesterol, Low Saturated Fat Diet. Retrieved February 16, 2020, from https://www.ucsfhealth.org/education/guidelines-for-a-low cholesterol-low-saturated-fat-diet

Wüest, F. (n.d.). 90% of People Quit After 3 Months of Hitting the Gym, Here's How to Be the Exception. Retrieved February 16, 2020, from https://www.lifehack.org/649556/90-of-people-quit-after-3-months-of-hitting-the-gym-heres-how-to-be-the-excep

www.ingramcontent.com/pod-product-compliance
Lightning Source LLC
Chambersburg PA
CBHW020417290526
45785CB00002B/597